Neural Nets in Electric Fish

Computational Neuroscience Series
Terrence J. Sejnowski and Tomaso A. Poggio, editors

Methods in Neuronal Modeling: From Synapses to Networks,
edited by Christof Koch and Idan Segev, 1989

Neural Nets in Electric Fish, Walter Heiligenberg, 1991

Neural Nets in Electric Fish

Walter Heiligenberg

A Bradford Book
The MIT Press
Cambridge, Massachusetts
London, England

This book was set in Trump Medieval by DEKR Corporation.

Library of Congress Cataloging-in-Publication Data

Heiligenberg, Walter, 1938-
  Neural nets in electric fish / Walter Heiligenberg.
    p. cm.—(Computational neuroscience)
  "A Bradford book."
  Includes bibliographical references and index.
  ISBN 978-0-262-08203-7 (hc.: alk. paper) — 978-0-262-51913-7 (pb. : alk. paper)
    1. Electroreceptors. 2. Jamming avoidance response (Electro-
physiology) 3. Neural circuitry. 4. Eigenmannia—Physiology.
  I. Title. II. Series.
QP447.5.H45   1991
597'.52—dc20   90-27589
                                                        CIP

MIT Press is pleased to keep this title available in print by manufacturing single copies,
on demand, via digital printing technology.

To Zsuzsa

Contents

Series Foreword

Computational neuroscience is an approach to understanding the information content of neural signals by modeling the nervous system at many different structural scales, including the biophysical, the circuit, and the systems levels. Computer simulations of neurons and neural networks are complementary to traditional techniques in neuroscience. This book series welcomes contributions that link theoretical studies with experimental approaches to understanding information processing in the nervous system. Areas and topics of particular interest include biophysical mechanisms for computation in neurons, computer simulations of neural circuits, models of learning, representation of sensory information in neural networks, systems models of sensory-motor integration, and computational analysis of problems in biological sensing, motor control, and perception.

Terrence J. Sejnowski
Tomaso Poggio

Foreword

This book is essentially about one behavior in one species, the jamming avoidance response in the electric fish *Eigenmannia*. It should, however, serve as a frame of reference for modelers and the students of other sensory systems. Computational neuroscience is a theory-rich and data-poor field, unlike some other branches of biology in which the opposite situation tends to prevail. The applicability of many computational models to the nervous system remains untested because so little is known about how real neural systems work. Many sensory networks are not amenable to systematic analysis of all stages of signal processing. This is the first vertebrate example in which the workings of the entire behavioral system from sensory input to motor output are almost completely understood.

What distinguishes this study from many other studies of sensory systems is its origins in the tradition of ethology. Heiligenberg was a student of the late Konrad Lorenz, one of the founding fathers of ethology. Neuroethology, which sprang from ethology, is the study of neural bases of natural behaviors such as swimming, singing, mating, prey capture, and predator evasion. The brain of an animal is designed to process biologically relevant stimuli and control behavior that is important for its survival and reproduction. This idea underlies all neuroethological studies and shapes the choice of animals and behavior, methods of study, collection of data, and interpretation of results. In this book, the reader can learn how neuroethologists think and work and how the significance of the story told here goes far beyond this special field into systems neurobiology in general and computational neuroscience in particular.

Heiligenberg and his associates began their study with the analysis of the behavior to define the problems that the animal's brain must solve. They studied the solution of the problems by modeling and tested the models in behavioral experiments. Their models predicted some of the neural mechanisms that were found later. They then studied how peripheral sensory neurons encode the stimulus that releases the behavior. The next step was to investigate where and how the primary sensory codes are used for the derivation of the codes for different features of the stimulus. In this way, they reached the brain area where neurons encode the stimulus that induces the jamming avoidance response. This behavior is now understood both at the level of algorithms and at that of neural implementation. This knowledge allows one to compare the operation of different behavioral systems. Such comparisons reveal remarkable similarities at the level of algorithms between different sensory systems and species of animals, suggesting the existence of general rules of signal processing.

This book is dedicated to Zsuzsa Heiligenberg, who saw it in the making but did not live to see it. This vivacious, charming, and cultured lady created a lively and interesting life, which fueled her husband's indefatigable spirit of investigation.

Mark Konishi
California Institute of Technology

Preface

This monograph attempts to explain the control of a specific behavior, the jamming avoidance response (JAR) of a weakly electric fish, on the basis of structural and functional properties of neuronal assemblies. After a brief introduction to the natural history of electric fish in chapter 2, behavioral properties of the JAR and experimental strategies for their analysis will be presented in chapter 3. The neuronal substrate of this behavior will be described in chapter 4, starting at the sensory input and progressing to the motor output. General issues, such as the nature of neuronal "feature detectors" and properties of a distributed neuronal organization of perception and motor control, will be discussed in chapter 5.

The neuronal analysis of the JAR began in Theodore H. Bullock's laboratory at Scripps Institution of Oceanography where I was introduced to this field upon joining his team in 1972. In addition to Theodore H. Bullock, a growing group of students, postdoctoral fellows, and visiting colleagues collaborated with me in further studies after my laboratory had been established at the same institution in 1973. In temporal order, these were Konstantin Behrend, Curtis Baker, Joanne Matsubara, Joseph Bastian, Carl Hopkins, Brian Partridge, John Harlan Meyer, Leonard Maler, Thomas Finger, Catherine Carr, Barbara Taylor, Gary Rose, Mary Hagedorn, Harold Zakon, John Dye, Caroly Shumway, Bruce Mathieson, Thomas Szabo, Clifford Keller, Günther Zupanc, Masashi Kawasaki, Heinrich Vischer, Walter Metzner, and Svenja Viete. For many years now, Grace Kennedy has run our histological projects with superb skills and devotion. My deepest thanks to all of them.

The first neuronal model of the JAR was developed by Scheich and Bullock (1974). Subsequent experiments by Heiligenberg, Baker and Matsubara (1978b), however, yielded results that were no longer compatible with the original model and suggested a very different neuronal organization, based on a distributed system of amplitude and phase computations and referred to as a "neuronal democracy." This new concept was further supported when subsequent experiments by Heiligenberg and Bastian (1980) employed an analog delay line to generate phase modulations in electric signals artificially. These modulations, although they do not occur naturally, caused behavioral effects that could be predicted by the new theory. On the basis of these findings, rigorous postulates could then be made about the neuronal substrate of the JAR, such as the existence of a circuit for the computation of temporal disparities, or differential phases, between signals at different points on the body surface. A long series of experiments, performed in collaboration with Bastian, Matsubara, Partridge, Carr, and Rose, then explored neuronal structures processing sensory information for the control of the JAR, and this work was reviewed by Heiligenberg in 1986. A major flaw in this latest presentation, the claim that the tectum opticum was required for the JAR, was corrected by Keller, Maler, and Heiligenberg (1990) in connection with their studies of the diencephalon. More recent studies, focusing on the control of the pacemaker frequency in connection with the JAR and social communication, have explored the organization and role of the diencephalic prepacemaker nucleus and of the medullary pacemaker nucleus. This latest work was performed in collaboration with Dye, Kawasaki, Keller, Maler, and Rose, and was briefly reviewed by Heiligenberg in 1989.

This work has been supported continually by grants from NSF, NIMH, and NINCDS. The National Geographic Society funded several excursions to the habitats of these fish in South and Central America. The Smithsonian Tropical Research Institute in Panama, the INPA in Manaus, Brasil, Dr. Horacio Vanegas at the IVIC Institute in Caracas, Venezuela, Dr. F. Mago-Leccia at the Instituto de

Zoologia Tropical in Caracas, and the Forest Service in Surinam generously offered use of their facilities. Again, my deepest thanks.

The writing of this monograph has benefited greatly from very critical comments and suggestions made by Theodore H. Bullock, John Dye, Carl Hopkins, Masashi Kawasaki, Clifford Keller, Gary Rose, and John Spiro. I am most grateful for their assistance.

Neural Nets in Electric Fish

1 Introduction

WHY STUDY ELECTRIC FISH?

Why should we explore exotic sensory systems such as electrosensation in fish or echolocation in bats? Is it only to satisfy the curiosity of comparative zoologists who are fascinated by the immense diversity of morphological and physiological adaptations to peculiar environments and ecological demands? Or is there reason to believe that the exploration of unusual and highly specialized sensory capabilities in other organisms might ultimately yield insight into the organization of our own brain?

More highly evolved organisms derive their superior qualities not so much from novel mechanisms at the cellular level but rather from a richer complexity in the orchestration of basic designs that they share with simpler organisms. Fundamental mechanisms of perception and neuronal processing of sensory information are shared by animals as diverse as flies and primates, but a larger number of neuronal structures and interconnecting pathways bestow more powerful computational abilities and memory capacities upon the brains of primates. Therefore, basic mechanisms of neuronal information processing may more profitably be studied in simpler organisms, as their brains are less complex and more amenable to experimentation. Much as genetic studies on simpler organisms have enabled us to understand the workings of our own genome, the exploration of simple brains should yield insight into the design of our own.

If it may now appear justifiable and even prudent to study, for example, vision in frogs, why then should we pay so much attention to sensory systems that humans do not share? The answer is that some animal species are champions in particular aspects of sensory or motor performance and that such superior capabilities are linked to highly specialized neuronal structures. Such structures incorporate and optimize particular neuronal designs that may be less conspicuous in organisms lacking these superior capabilities. Moreover, the behavioral repertoire of such "champion" species readily offers paradigms for testing the performance of their special designs at the level of the intact animal. Electric fish and echolocating bats, for example, are masters in the processing of temporal information and show an abundance of mechanisms devoted to the analysis of temporal signal characteristics. Therefore, these animals provide powerful model systems for behavioral as well as cellular studies of a wide scope of neural mechanisms dedicated to temporal information processing. Their exploration will reveal the diversity and limitations of these mechanisms and should ultimately facilitate our understanding of temporal information processing in other systems, for example, speech perception in humans.

EXPERIMENTAL STRATEGIES

The study of brain mechanisms requires thorough knowledge of the animal's sensory and behavioral capabilities. Animals are naturally adapted to detect and to process very specific stimulus patterns in their environment, and studies of their ecology and ethology help us to identify these relevant stimulus patterns as well as the natural behavioral responses that they evoke and control. Since we cannot interrogate animals as we do human subjects in psychophysical tests, these responses provide crucial assays for the experimental dissection of stimulus patterns and for the identification of their critical components. Moreover, experimental manipulation of these components and their configuration in stimulus patterns enable us to pin down the computational rules that underlie the evaluation of patterns by the animal's brain. In the course of this analysis, we gain confidence in our conceptual models of perception to the extent that we are able to predict behavioral consequences that are due to specific alterations in stimulus patterns.

After behavioral experiments have identified computational rules of perception, their specific neuronal implementations can be determined by physiological and anatomical approaches. The overwhelming structural and functional complexities of brain mechanisms motivate us to study neuronal mechanisms in the relatively simple systems found in invertebrates and lower vertebrates, such as fish and amphibians. The small size of their brains as well as the more modest number of structural components and interconnections facilitate analysis at the single-cell level.

The electrosensory system of certain orders of fish appears to have a relatively simple structural and functional organization, but it also displays sophisticated features, such as complex receptive fields, ordered central representations, and modulations of sensory processing by recurrent descending pathways. Such features are known to occur in more advanced sensory systems, such as mammalian vision and hearing. What make the electrosensory system particularly appealing are behavioral responses, such as the jamming avoidance response (JAR), that remain intact in physiological preparations. Studies at the single-cell level can thus be combined with simultaneous behavioral assays to test the significance of stimulus patterns for both the cell and the whole animal as well as to monitor the overall intactness of the system during experiments.

In the case of the JAR, the intactness of the behavior has been found to be a crucial condition for the exploration of higher-order neurons. Without obvious signs of physical stress or general deterioration of vegetative functions, an animal may gradually cease to respond to stimulus patterns that normally elicit and control this behavior. And higher-order neurons that are known to discriminate such patterns fail to do so as the animal ceases to respond. While that should not be surprising, traditionally most neurophysiological studies have been performed without observing concurrent behavioral responses. It is highly questionable how much can be learned about the functions of single neurons by studying anesthetized, nonbehaving animals.

The following presentation will begin with a brief introduction to the natural history of electric fish, followed by a detailed description of a specific behavioral phenomenon, the JAR of the weakly electric fish *Eigenmannia*. This has become a valuable model system for the exploration of neuronal mechanisms of sensory information processing. My description will emphasize how the experimental analysis of stimulus patterns controlling the JAR leads us to postulate particular computational mechanisms at the neuronal level. The physiology and anatomy of these mechanisms will then be presented by tracing the flow of information from the receptor level to the ultimate control of the motor pattern. A detailed review of electrosensation was recently edited by Bullock and Heiligenberg (1986), and the reader may turn to this volume for a more exhaustive treatment of issues that are outside the focus of this presentation.

2 The Behavior and Ecology of Electric Fish

Gymnotiform fishes of South America and mormyriform fishes of Africa generate electric fields by discharging an electric organ in the tail section of their body. Arrays of electroreceptors on the body surface detect the fish's own field as well as fields of neighbors. Objects differing in their impedance from the surrounding water distort the animal's field (figure 2.1), and the pattern of distortions on the body surface represents the electric image of such objects. Electric fish are able to assess their environment by analyzing electric images, and this "electrolocation" (Lissmann 1958, Lissmann and Machin 1958) of objects can, therefore, be considered a form of "seeing" with the body surface (Bullock 1968).

Two principal aspects of the electric signal associated with the fish's electric organ discharge (EOD) are affected by nearby objects. These are the local amplitude of the signal and its phase, that is, the timing of its zero-crossing. The modulations shown in figure 2.2 have been exaggerated for demonstration purposes. Natural forms of object-induced modulations are shown in figure 2.3. Amplitude and phase are coded by separate sets of receptors, which will be described in chapter 4.

By monitoring the EODs of neighbors and by modulating their own discharges in accordance with particular behavioral states and intentions, electric fish communicate in the context of territorial and reproductive behavior (Hopkins 1972, 1974a,b,c; Hagedorn and Heiligenberg 1985, see reviews by Hagedorn 1986, Hopkins 1986, 1988). Electric fish produce species-typical EOD signals (figure 2.4), and while *wave-species* generate continuous, nearly sinusoidal

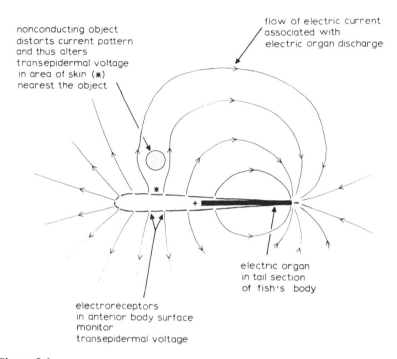

nonconducting object distorts current pattern and thus alters transepidermal voltage in area of skin (✳) nearest the object

flow of electric current associated with electric organ discharge

electric organ in tail section of fish's body

electroreceptors in anterior body surface monitor transepidermal voltage

Figure 2.1
The principle of electrolocation. In this horizontal section through a simplified electric fish, the black bar indicates the location of the electric organ. This organ is discharged at a regular rate under the command of the pacemaker nucleus in the fish's hindbrain (not shown). Electroreceptors are found in pores of the body surface, and their density is highest in the rostral region. The interior of the body is of relatively low resistance, while the resistance of the skin is high and forces current to flow through the pores occupied by electroreceptors. Internal shunting of current is prevented by insulating tissue that wraps the electric organ and surrounds it tightly within the narrow tail filament. An object with an impedance different from that of the surrounding water will alter the pattern of transepidermal voltage, and this alteration represents the electric image of the object. (From Heiligenberg 1977a)

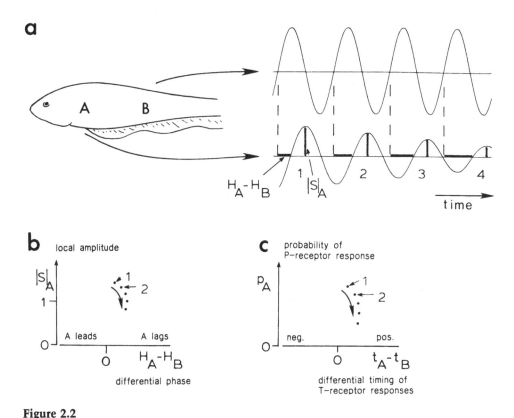

Figure 2.2
Objects in the vicinity of the animal's body surface may locally alter the electric signal
generated by the animal's EOD in two ways, causing a change in amplitude (|S|) and a
shift in phase (H). (a) The EOD is idealized as a sinusoidal signal and is recorded as
voltage in locations A and B, respectively. The signal in location A is assumed to be
distorted by the passage of a small object, whereas the signal in location B is undis-
turbed. As the object passes location A, the local amplitude of the signal (|S|$_A$) is
gradually attenuated, while the "differential phase" (H$_A$–H$_B$), measured as the difference in the timing of the zero-crossings of the signals in A and B, increases progressively. The sizes of the modulations in amplitude and phase have been exaggerated for
purpose of illustration. In the absence of the perturbation in A, the differential phase
(H$_A$–H$_B$) would be zero. (b) As successive pairs of values of |S|$_A$ and H$_A$–H$_B$, sampled
for successive cycles, 1,2,3, . . . , are plotted in a two-dimensional plane, a graph is
obtained which reflects the motion of the object. As will be explained later in detail,
the information plotted in the two-dimensional plane in (b) is coded by two classes of
electroreceptors (c). The probability (p$_A$) of P-type receptor firing in location A reflects
the value of the local amplitude. T-type receptors fire one spike on each EOD cycle
and at a fixed latency with reference to the timing of the local zero-crossing. The
difference in timing of T-type action potentials in A and B, t$_A$–t$_B$, therefore, reflects
the differential phase, H$_A$–H$_B$.

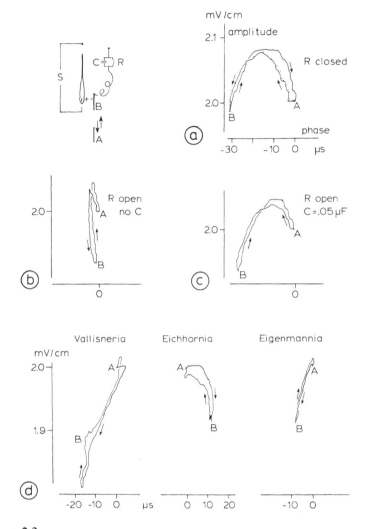

Figure 2.3
An object causes local modulations in the amplitude and the phase of the current associated with the fish's EOD; the nature of these modulations depends on the electrical qualities of the object as well as on the direction of its motion. The inset in the upper left is a top view of a fish temporarily immobilized by injection of a curarelike drug. Since this drug also silences the animal's EOD, a substitute signal, S, of similar frequency (500 Hz), amplitude, and field geometry is provided by a signal generator and electrodes placed inside the mouth and at the tip of the tail. The EOD-like signal is recorded by a pair of differential electrodes (+ −) at the side of the animal's head. An object is moved sinusoidally at a rate of 0.5 Hz back and forth between the locations A and B, approximately 1 cm away from and parallel to the animal's body surface. In (a) to (d), the local peak-to-peak amplitude of S is plotted on the ordinate, while its phase (i.e., its zero-

EODs, *pulse-species* emit individual pulses separated by longer intervals of silence. Wave-type fish fire their electric organ at very stable, though individually distinct, fundamental frequencies within a species-typical range that may be as low as 50 to 100 Hz in the gymnotiform genus *Sternopygus* and higher than 1000 Hz in the related genus *Apteronotus* (figure 2.5). Pulse-type fish emit pulses of a species-typical shape and duration at a rather variable repetition rate in the range of a few to well over one hundred per second. The duration of a pulse may be as short as a few tenths of a millisecond in one mormyrid species and as long as several milliseconds in another species (figure 2.6). EOD frequencies and waveforms may show a sexual difference during the reproductive season and subserve sexual recognition (Hopkins 1980, 1988; Bass and Hopkins 1983, 1985; figure 2.7).

The absence of EOD forms intermediate between continuous, wavelike signals and discrete, pulselike signals suggests that the two types of EODs convey particular and incompatible advantages. Yet, so far there is no evidence that wave-type and pulse-type EODs are adapted to particular forms of electrolocation. As will be shown below, however, they allow for different mechanisms to avoid jamming by EODs of neighbors.

---

crossing), measured in microseconds and in reference to the cycle of the signal generator, is plotted on the abscissa. Since the frequency of S is 500 Hz, a full cycle (i.e., a phase value of 2π) measures 2 ms. A signal amplitude of 2 mV/cm and a phase defined as zero are recorded with the object in position A, which is distant from the animal. In (a) to (c), the object is a thin, 1.5 cm wide, vertically suspended strip of metal foil, insulated on the side facing away from the animal. This foil is connected via a capacitor (C) or an electrical short (R closed) to a distant point in the water. In (a), dots mark every tenth cycle of the EOD-like signal, S, as the object travels from A to B. Arrows indicate the direction of motion in the amplitude-phase plane. Although the physical motion from A to B is, theoretically, symmetrical to the motion from B to A, slight turbulence-related asymmetries in the motion cause differences in the respective sections of the graph. Different natural objects were chosen in (d), a leaf of the water plant *Vallisneria*, approximately 1.5 cm wide; a bulbous leaf stem of the water hyacinth, *Eichhornia*, approximately 2 cm in diameter; and a conspecific fish, with its EOD silenced by MS222 anesthesia to avoid electrical interference. (From Rose and Heiligenberg 1986a)

MORMYRIFORMS

family	genus	EOD pulse- or wave mode	general appearance
MORMYRIDAE			
	Mormyrus	p	
	Gnathonemus	p	
	Brienomyrus	p	
	Pollimyrus	p	
GYMNARCHIDAE			
	Gymnarchus	w (250-500 Hz)	

GYMNOTIFORMS

family	genus	EOD	general appearance
GYMNOTIDAE			
	Gymnotus	p	
ELECTROPHORIDAE			
	Electrophorus	p	
HYPOPOMIDAE			
	Hypopomus	p	
	Parupygus	p	
	Hypopygus	p	
	Steatogenys	p	
RHAMPHICHTHYIDAE			
	Rhamphichthys	p	
	Gymnorhamphichthys	p	
STERNOPYGIDAE			
	Sternopygus	w (50-200 Hz)	
	Rhabdolichops	w (600-900 Hz)	
	Eigenmannia	w (200-500 Hz)	
APTERONOTIDAE			
	Apteronotus	w (700-1000 Hz)	
	Adontosternarchus	w (700-1250 Hz)	
	Sternarchorhamphus	w (700-1000 Hz)	
	Sternarchorhynchus	w (1500-1800 Hz)	

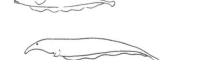

EVOLUTIONARY AND ECOLOGICAL CONSIDERATIONS

Wave-type and pulse-type EODs have evolved in gymnotiforms as well as in mormyriforms, two relatively unrelated orders that most likely invented electroreception and electrogenesis independently. This view, originally suggested on the basis of taxonomic considerations, is strongly supported by distinct differences in the central electrosensory pathways of these two orders (Finger et al. 1986). Although all ancestral forms of fishes appear to have been electroreceptive, this sensory modality was lost with the evolution of the teleost fishes. The loss of this modality is as much a puzzle as is its reappearance within a few isolated groups of teleosts (Northcutt 1986).

The original type of electroreceptors are *ampullary* organs of the Lorenzinian kind and are most sensitive to low-frequency signals below 40 Hz. These organs, known as "ampullae of Lorenzini" in sharks and rays, are found in all ancestral forms of fishes except hagfish (myxinoids). A quite different kind of ampullary organ newly evolved at least twice in the electrosensitive teleosts, the mormyriforms, the Notopterinae (a subfamily of African knife fish, related to the mormyriforms), the gymnotiforms, and the siluriforms (catfish). Ampullary organs detect weak electric fields of geophysical, chemical, or biological origin. They enable fish to orient and navigate with reference to large-scale fields in oceans and river

Figure 2.4
Families and most common genera of electric fish. Drawings roughly indicate relative sizes of fish. Maximal adult lengths are: 10–30 cm for mormyrids, more than 1 m for *Gymnarchus*, 50–80 cm for *Gymnotus*, 20–30 cm for Apteronotids. All species live in fresh water of the tropics, the mormyriforms in Africa and the gymnotiforms in South and Central America. In all families, with the exception of Apteronotids, the electric organ is "myogenic," i.e., derived from skeletal musculature. The "neurogenic" electric organ of Apteronotids is derived from the axons of spinal motor neurons, which must have innervated a myogenic electric organ in their ancestors (Bennett 1971, Waxman et al. 1972, see review by Bass 1986). A myogenic organ is still found in the juvenile forms of Apteronotids but is then abandoned as the adult, neurogenic organ develops (Kirschbaum 1983). In contrast to myogenic organs, neurogenic organs cannot be silenced by injection of curarelike drugs, which block acetylcholine receptors. The classification of gymnotiform families was adopted from Mago-Leccia (1978). Complete lists of mormyrids and gymnotiforms have been compiled by Hopkins (1986, 1988).

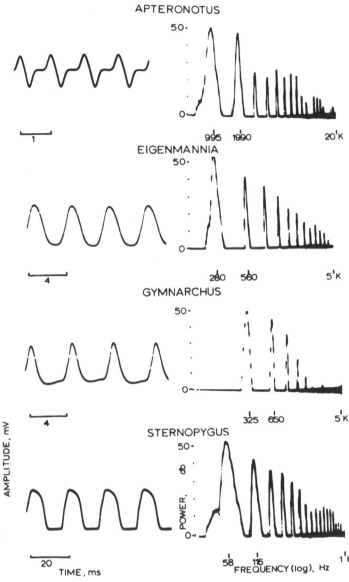

Figure 2.5
EODs and the corresponding power spectra of representative wave-type species. EODs were recorded with a positive electrode in front of the head and a negative electrode behind the tip of the tail. The input resistance of the differential amplifier was above 1 MΩ, and the resistivity of the water was several kΩm·cm. Amplitude spectra were obtained by fast Fourier analysis of digitized EOD samples. (From Bullock et al. 1975)

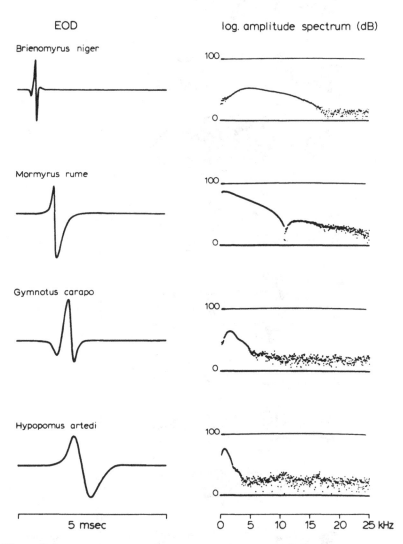

Figure 2.6
EODs of representative pulse-type species. Recordings and presentation as
in figure 2.5. Amplitude spectra were calculated by transient capture Fourier analysis of a single discharge. The species name, *Hypopomus artedi*,
was chosen incorrectly in earlier publications and should be replaced by
the name *Hypopomus brevirostris*. (From Heiligenberg 1977a)

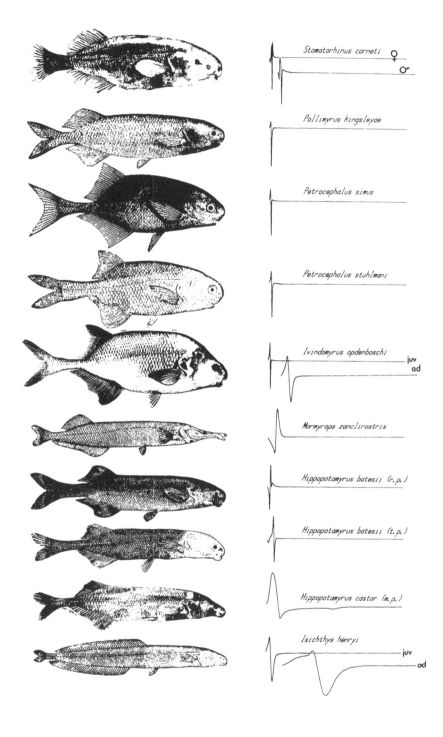

Stomatorhinus corneti ♀
♂

Pollimyrus kingsleyae

Petrocephalus simus

Petrocephalus stuhlmani

Ivindomyrus opdenboschi   juv
ad

Mormyrops zanclirostris

Hippopotamyrus batesii (r.p.)

Hippopotamyrus batesii (t.p.)

Hippopotamyrus castor (m.p.)

Isichthys henryi   juv
ad

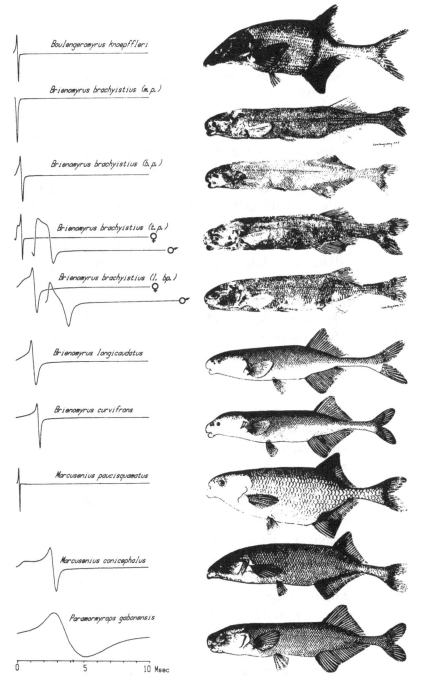

Figure 2.7
Sympatric species of mormyrids of the Ivindo River in Gabon. The wave-
form of their EODs serves in sex and species recognition. (Courtesy of C.
D. Hopkins)

systems, as well as to detect prey on the basis of small, local fields emanating from living tissue underwater (see reviews by Kalmijn 1984, 1987).

An additional class of electroreceptors, known as the *tuberous* organs, is found in the mormyriforms and gymnotiforms, which, in addition, have independently evolved electric organs from muscle or nerve tissue to generate electric fields actively. Tuberous organs are most sensitive in the range of the dominant spectral frequencies of the animal's EODs (Hopkins 1976) and serve in electrolocation and communication. Mormyriforms and gymnotiforms thus have two kinds of electric senses adapted to different functions, and, as will be shown later, their central representations are separate across several synaptic levels. Different subtypes of tuberous organs are adapted to encode specific signal parameters, such as amplitude or phase of a sinusoidal EOD, or to discriminate between signals of different amplitude, such as the animal's own EODs and the EODs of distant neighbors. As will be shown later, this differentiation of receptor subtypes enhances the animal's resolution of electric details in its environment (see review by Zakon 1986).

The evolution of electrolocation and electrical communication has helped mormyriforms and gymnotiforms to live nocturnally and in waters of poor visibility. As a consequence, they are relatively safe from visual predators and can exploit food sources that remain hidden for other orders of fish. Much as bats were able to invade new ecological niches by the invention of sonar, electric fish have assumed a dominant role in the nightly waters of the tropics by exploiting electrical cues. However, in contrast to sonar, the use of EODs is limited to short distances. The electric field generated by a fish's EODs is similar to that produced by a dipole. At distances of more than a few body lengths, that is, several dipole lengths, the magnitude of the EOD field potential, therefore, falls off as the second power of the distance from the source, while the magnitude of the spatial voltage gradient attenuates as the third power. In order to travel more than a few meters from their individual daytime hiding places, electric fish therefore may have to rely on memory, much as a blind man feeling his way across town.

NOISE AND SIGNAL INTERFERENCE

Lightning generates electrical pulses and oscillations that propagate over hundreds of kilometers through tropical waters and easily surpass the detection thresholds of tuberous organs (Hopkins 1973). While narrow tuning of electroreceptors to the dominant spectral frequency or the pulse shape of the animal's own EOD may provide some protection against noise related to lightning, electric fish achieve additional immunity by firing EODs repetitively and focusing on features represented consistently across several successive EODs (Heiligenberg 1976). They are thus less vulnerable to the singular and erratic perturbations caused by this kind of environmental noise. A more serious source of interference are the EODs of conspecifics that approximately match the animal's own peripheral and central sensory filter characteristics. Different mechanisms have evolved to cope with this form of jamming.

Behavioral experiments have shown that the ability of *pulse-type species* to electrolocate objects is most vulnerable to pulses coinciding with the animal's own EODs, particularly if several successive EODs are hit by coincidences (Heiligenberg 1974, 1976). Gymnotiform pulse-species produce EODs at rather regular rates, and successive coincidences only occur when two animals have very similar EOD rates. These fish minimize the chance of successive coincidences by slightly modulating their pulse rates whenever their EODs drift toward each other in time and collisions are imminent (Heiligenberg 1977a, Scheich et al. 1977, Heiligenberg et al. 1978a). Whereas the role of electroreceptors has been studied in great detail by Baker (1980, 1981), little is yet known about central neuronal mechanisms underlying this form of jamming avoidance behavior.

All known mormyrids (see figure 2.4) emit pulselike EODs at rather irregular intervals. This, as well as the extremely small width of EOD pulses typical for gregarious species (Hopkins 1980), makes successive coincidences between EODs of neighbors very unlikely. At high EOD rates, however, mormyrids too fire at more regular intervals (Moller 1970). Individuals can minimize the chance of pulse coincidences by discharging at a specific, short latency with reference to the neighbor's most recent EOD and thus hitting a moment in time when their neighbor is least likely to fire (Bell et al. 1974, Kramer 1974, Heiligenberg 1977a).

Coincidences cannot be avoided in the case of continuous, wave-like EODs. Behavioral experiments have shown that the ability of *wave-type species* to electrolocate is most vulnerable to signal frequencies near the animal's own EOD fundamental (Heiligenberg 1973, 1975, 1977a). All species tested so far, with the exception of the gymnotiform genus *Sternopygus*, avoid this form of jamming by shifting their EOD frequencies in an apparent effort to increase the frequency difference between the interfering EODs (Watanabe and Takeda 1963, Bullock et al. 1972). This jamming avoidance response (JAR) is quite robust and still functions in animals temporarily immobilized by the injection of curarelike drugs, which greatly facilitates physiological studies of neural structures participating in the control of this behavior (Scheich and Bullock 1974). A multitude of behavioral experiments have determined the computational rules that guide the perception of stimulus patterns eliciting this form of JAR in the gymnotiform genus *Eigenmannia*, and the same rules were later found to hold for a related genus, *Apteronotus*, as well (Heiligenberg 1986).

The discovery of the computational rules guiding the JAR of *Eigenmannia* will be presented in chapter 3. It will be shown how the experimental dissection of a stimulus complexity identifies a perceptual space with two orthogonal parameters, amplitude and phase. Moreover, one can demonstrate that this perceptual space matches specific computational operations that are executed in the central nervous system. The neuronal implementation of these operations will be presented in chapter 4.

3 The Jamming Avoidance Response of *Eigenmannia*

THE EXPERIMENTAL OPENING OF A LOOP

Electric organs of the mormyriform and gymnotiform fishes have originated from skeletal muscles. Only in a single and apparently most advanced family of gymnotiforms, the Apteronotidae (see figure 2.4), has the role of the myogenic electric organ been taken over by its highly modified spinal innervation, and these neurogenic electric organs are capable of firing at much higher frequencies than the myogenic organs of all other families (Bennett 1971, see review by Bass 1986). The evolutionary transformation from a myogenic to a neurogenic organ appears to be recapitulated in the larval development of apteronotid fish (Kirschbaum 1983).

Myogenic organs are activated by the transmitter acetylcholine, as are muscles, and consequently these organs can be silenced by drugs, such as curare, that block cholinergic transmission. Silencing the electric organ, however, does not interfere with the regular discharge activity of the pacemaker in the animal's hindbrain, which drives the electric organ by triggering each discharge by a single command pulse (figure 3.1). By monitoring the activity of the pacemaker or the spinal volley associated with each command pulse, one can, therefore, determine the intended activity of the electric organ. In particular, any effort of the immobilized animal to change its would-be electric organ discharge (EOD) frequency can be monitored in this way.

The tuberous electroreceptors on the animal's body surface are driven predominantly by the animal's own EOD current. The relatively weak currents associated with the EODs of neighbors only modulate the effect of this dominant signal. After the electric organ

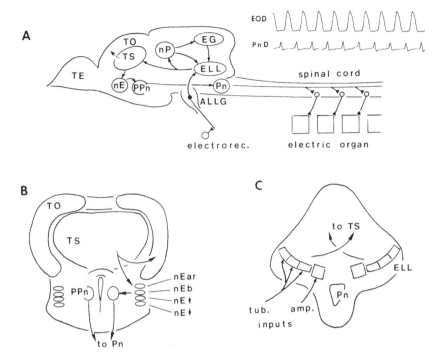

Figure 3.1
Sketches of neural structures and pathways involved in the JAR and other
electrosensory behaviors. More details will be given in figure 4.52. A longitudinal section is shown in (A), and transverse sections at the levels of
the midbrain/diencephalon and hindbrain are shown in (B) and (C), respectively. (A): Primary afferent neurons in the anterior lateral line nerve ganglion (ALLG) relay information from electroreceptors on the body surface
to the electrosensory lateral line lobe (ELL) in the hindbrain. The ELL
projects to the torus semicircularis (TS) of the midbrain, and collaterals of
neurons coding amplitude information also project to the nucleus praeeminentialis (nP). The nP, in turn, is a source of two descending inputs to the
ELL, one direct and one indirect via the eminentia granularis (EG) of the
cerebellum. The TS projects to the tectum opticum (TO) and to nucleus
electrosensorius (nE) of the diencephalon, which appears to drive the prepacemaker nucleus (PPn). The PPn, in turn, induces frequency modulations
of the pacemaker nucleus (Pn) in the medulla. The Pn innervates spinal
motor neurons which, in turn, innervate the electrocytes of the electric
organ. The inset in the upper right shows how each discharge of the electric
organ (EOD) is triggered by a single command pulse (PnD) from the Pn.
The EOD rate is 300 Hz. The TO as well as the telencephalon (TE) is not
required for the JAR. The transverse section in (B) shows that the nE is
composed of at least four subterritories, apparently dedicated to different
behavioral functions, and that the TS innervates both the nE complex and
the TO. The transverse section in (C) displays the three maps of the ELL
receiving identical input from tuberous electroreceptors, and the single
map receiving input from ampullary electroreceptors. The Pn is an unpaired
nucleus in the medulla.

has been silenced experimentally, the effect of the animal's own EODs as well as that of interfering EODs can be simulated electronically, thus giving the experimenter complete control over the electrosensory information (Scheich and Bullock 1974). This capacity to substitute natural stimulus patterns by specific mimics as well as to record intact behavioral responses in an immobilized animal has been instrumental in the study of the neuronal organization underlying the jamming avoidance response (JAR).

(To perform similar experiments on apteronotid fish, which have neurogenic electric organs and, therefore, cannot be silenced by curarization, one is forced to eliminate EODs through spinal transection. An EOD mimic can then be offered much as in the case of *Eigenmannia*, and the pacemaker frequency can be monitored by recording directly from the medullary pacemaker nucleus. Unpublished experiments of this kind revealed no basic differences in the organization of the JAR of *Eigenmannia* and that of members of the apteronotid family.)

BEHAVIORAL RULES FOR THE JAR

After Watanabe and Takeda (1963) discovered that gymnotiform species with wave-type EODs were capable of shifting their EOD frequency away from similar interfering frequencies, Bullock and his collaborators set out to study the dynamics and organization of this behavioral response. Assuming that these fish required a private and undisturbed frequency band for proper electrolocation of objects, they called this behavior *jamming avoidance response* (Bullock et al. 1972). Behavioral measurements of the acuity of electrolocation then demonstrated that interfering signals at frequencies similar to that of the animal's own EODs indeed impair electrolocation performance in *Eigenmannia* (Heiligenberg 1973), while the genus *Sternopygus*, which alone does not have a JAR (Bullock et al. 1972), is immune to jamming as long as stimulus intensities do not exceed their natural range (Matsubara and Heiligenberg 1978).

The fish discriminates sign and magnitude of the frequency difference between the jamming signal and its EOD

Eigenmannia lowers its EOD frequency in response to jamming signals of slightly higher frequency and raises its EOD frequency in response to signals of slightly lower frequency. Sinusoidal jamming signals can readily be produced with a function generator, and by clamping the frequency of this generator with respect to the EOD frequency of the fish, a constant frequency difference (Df) can be maintained between the two signals regardless of any EOD frequency shifts produced by the fish. By choosing a given magnitude of Df and switching its sign at regular intervals, the fish's EOD frequency can be driven up and down indefinitely. The largest responses are obtained for magnitudes of Df in the range of 2 to 6 Hz (Bullock et al. 1972). The same range of Dfs was also found to be most detrimental for electrolocation performance (Matsubara and Heiligenberg 1978 in *Eigenmannia*, and similar unpublished behavioral observations on the apterontid genus *Adontosternarchus*. Neuronal data by Behrend 1977).

When a fish is suddenly exposed to a jamming stimulus it may, as if startled, shift its frequency initially in a direction not related to the sign of the Df (Heiligenberg 1977a, Dye 1987). Following this transient response, as the fish is subjected to an ongoing jamming regimen, it shifts its EOD frequency always in the correct direction and responds with a latency of a few hundred milliseconds to the sudden switch of the sign of Df. Therefore, the fish is able to determine the sign of Df almost instantly and without "hunting" (Bullock et al. 1972). Which cues could the animal exploit to perform this task? Since the animal is capable of discriminating the sign of Df, one might assume that it is also able to identify which of the two interfering signal frequencies is its own.

The fish determines the sign of Df without internal reference to its pacemaker

Studies of the JAR have taught us that animals, in the course of their evolution, have not always opted for solutions that human engineers would consider optimal. Since the animal generates its own EOD frequency in the medullary pacemaker nucleus it could, in theory, identify its own EOD frequency simply by internal reference to its pacemaker. However, this hypothesis is ruled out by two kinds of experiments.

The first evidence against an internal reference to the pacemaker was provided by Bullock et al. (1972), who placed a fish into a two-compartment chamber and fitted an electrically tight seal around the pectoral region of the fish so that practically no EOD signal could any longer be detected at its head surface. Presentation of a jamming stimulus to the head alone failed to elicit a JAR in this case. Yet, to the extent that either the jamming signal was allowed to leak into the chamber containing the trunk, or the EOD signal was allowed to leak into the chamber containing the head, a JAR was evoked. This experiment thus demonstrated unambiguously that the fish needs to be exposed to the mixture of the two signals in some part of its body surface in order to execute a JAR.

Another experiment demonstrates directly that the fish does not use information that could be provided internally by its pacemaker. After the fish's EOD is silenced by curarization, an EOD mimic of similar amplitude and frequency can be provided electronically by placing one electrode in the fish's mouth and one at the tip of the tail (figure 3.2). This arrangement of electrodes results in an electric field geometry similar to that of the natural EOD. The EOD of a neighbor can then be mimicked by a pair of external electrodes straddling the fish. Under these conditions, the fish will execute a correct JAR by lowering its pacemaker frequency when the mimic of a neighbor's EOD has a frequency slightly higher than the mimic of its own EOD (i.e., when Df is positive), and it will raise its pacemaker frequency when Df is negative. Most importantly, however, the frequency of the animal's EOD mimic need not agree with its pacemaker frequency. Indeed, it may differ from its pacemaker frequency by as much as 100 Hz or more in either direction (Heiligenberg et al. 1978b).

(Still larger differences between the pacemaker frequency and the frequency of the EOD mimic will result in increasingly weaker behavioral responses. Since the tuberous electroreceptors are tuned

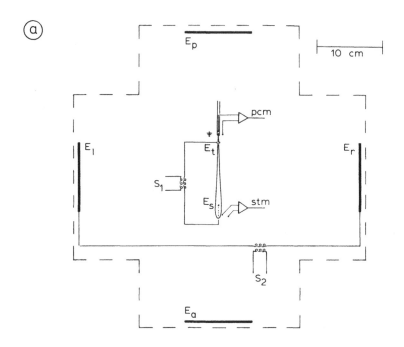

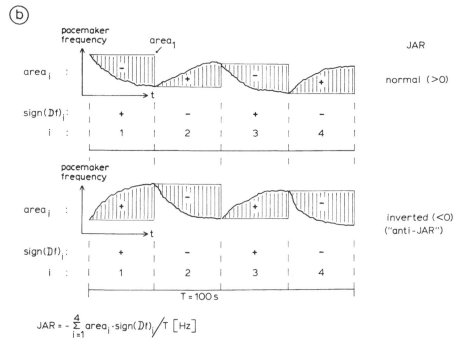

$$JAR = -\sum_{i=1}^{4} area_i \cdot sign(Df)_i \Big/ T \; [Hz]$$

to the fish's natural EOD frequency, they cannot be recruited sufficiently by signal frequencies too different from this frequency.
Tuberous electroreceptors thus represent bandpass filters, and stimulus patterns will drive the JAR to the extent that their frequencies
match the tuning of the fish's receptors [Kramer 1985].)

**The sign of Df is extracted from phase and amplitude information contained
in the interference pattern**

The experiments in figure 3.2 demonstrated that the fish discriminates the sign of Df by evaluating afferent information contained
in the interference, or "beat" pattern, which results from the mixing
of its own EOD with that of a neighbor. JARs can be elicited after
replacing the animal's own EOD as well as that of a potential
neighbor by pure sine waves. Contrary to earlier claims by Scheich
and Bullock (1974), the addition of higher-harmonic components,
which are required to approximate the natural EOD waveform, has
no detectable qualitative or quantitative consequences on the JAR,
as long as the two interfering EOD fields are provided through
separate pairs of electrodes so that the two fields have different

Figure 3.2
(a) The JAR can be elicited in a curarized fish after its silenced EOD has been replaced
by a sinusoidal substitute (S₁) of a similar frequency and amplitude, applied between
an electrode E_s in the fish's mouth and an electrode E_t at the tip of its tail. Due to the
internal location of E_s, the geometry of the S₁ current field resembles that of the fish's
natural EOD field. An electric stimulus (S₂) simulating the EOD field of a neighbor
can be applied either transversely, through electrodes E_l and E_r, or longitudinally,
through electrodes E_a and E_p. The intensity of either stimulus is measured by a pair
of electrodes placed near and perpendicular to the surface of the head (stm). The
pacemaker frequency is monitored by recording the spinal volley through a suction
electrode placed over the tip of the tail (pcm). (b) A JAR is elicited by switching the
sign of the Df between S₂ and S₁ every 25 s, with Df defined as positive if the frequency
of S₂ is higher than that of S₁. A magnitude of Df between 2 and 6 Hz is most effective.
The JAR is measured by adding the shaded areas, which represent integrated shifts in
pacemaker frequency from the most recent switch of the sign of Df. Downward shifts
are counted negatively, upward shifts positively (see signs inside shaded areas). The
formula shown at the bottom gives a positive value if the animal shows a correct JAR,
i.e., if it lowers its pacemaker frequency for positive Dfs and raises it for negative Dfs.
Wrong frequency shifts ("anti-JARs"), which can be elicited by certain stimulus configurations, yield a negative value. The JAR measure defined in this manner gives the
mean frequency shift over the whole period of stimulation, T. (From Heiligenberg et
al. 1978b)

geometries (Heiligenberg et al. 1978b). As a consequence of the ensuing difference in the current paths of the two fields, the mixing ratio of the two signals varies across the animal's body surface. If the two EOD stimuli are added electronically and their sum is then presented through the same pair of electrodes, however, JARs can no longer be elicited. Under this "identical geometry" condition, the two EOD fields, while differing in frequency, are spatially identical, and the mixing ratio of the two currents no longer varies across the animal's body surface.

This finding suggests the following mechanism for discriminating the sign of Df. Let the fish's own EOD or its substitute be represented by a sine wave stimulus S_1 and that of its neighbor by a sine wave stimulus S_2. Since S_1 originates from an internal current source it should recruit all electroreceptors on the animal's body surface evenly and at nearly the same phase of the stimulus cycle. Since S_2 originates from external sources, however, it will affect only some areas of the animal's body surface and will fail to drive receptors in those areas where its current flows parallel to the skin surface (figure 3.3). Since a neighbor is usually at some distance, the amplitude of S_2 should be smaller than that of S_1 at every point of the animal's body surface. As shown in figures 3.3 and 3.4, the mixing of S_1 and of an S_2 of smaller amplitude causes a modulation of the amplitude as well as of the phase of the mixed signal in reference to the pure S_1 signal or even in reference to another mixture of S_1 and S_2 with a still smaller contribution of S_2. If amplitude and phase values are recorded for successive S_1 cycles and then plotted in a two-dimensional, amplitude-versus-phase plane, a circular trajectory, or graph, is obtained that repeats itself at a rate equal to the magnitude of the difference of the two interfering frequencies, also referred to as "beat frequency." And the sense of rotation reflects the sign of the frequency difference: clockwise for negative Dfs, namely, when the frequency of S_2 is lower, and counterclockwise in the opposite case. Thus, if S_1 had a frequency of 400 Hz and S_2 had a frequency of 402 Hz, the amplitude-versus-phase plot would define a circular trajectory that would rotate counterclockwise and would complete two full cycles per

second. If *Eigenmannia* could determine the direction of rotation
in this graph, it could immediately gauge the direction of the necessary behavioral response. It should raise its frequency for clockwise rotations and lower its frequency for counterclockwise
rotations.

(Theoretically, the animal could also discriminate the sign of Df
by comparing amplitude modulations with modulations in instantaneous frequency, that is, the inverse of successive cycles of the
mixed signal. Plots of these two variables also yield circular graphs
with the direction of rotation reflecting the sign of Df [Heiligenberg
1977a]. That the animal does not use this information is shown by
the failure of the identical-geometry condition to elicit a JAR. This
condition only eliminates modulations in differential phase but
leaves modulations in instantaneous frequency intact.)

The computation of differential-phase information

Analysis of phase modulations requires that the animal have a
reference signal somewhere on its body surface. This could be a
pure S_1 sampled from an area of the body surface that is free from
S_2 interference, and the animal could identify such an area by the
local absence of amplitude modulations. However, one can demonstrate that the animal is still able to solve the problem even if
no pure representation of S_1 is available anywhere. This condition
can be obtained by electronically adding an attenuated representation of S_2 to S_1, while the regular S_2 is still being applied through
separate electrodes. This experiment shows that the JAR requires
nothing more than that some areas of the body surface be more
heavily contaminated by S_2 than others. How then does the animal
exploit information from differentially contaminated areas of its
body surface to discriminate the sign of Df?

The diagram in figure 3.5 addresses this question. Assume that
area A is more heavily contaminated by S_2 than area B and that the
angles formed by the S_1 and S_2 current vectors in A and B are both
either acute or obtuse at any moment. As a consequence of this
latter condition, the mixed signals in A and B will reach their peak
amplitudes always in synchrony. If one plots the local stimulus

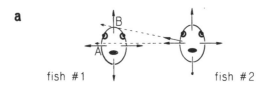

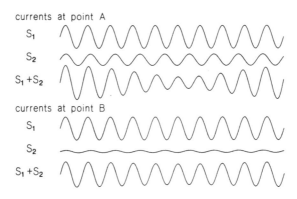

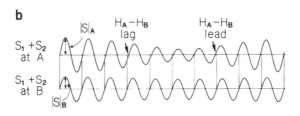

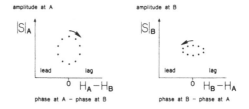

Figure 3.3

(a) The addition of the EOD currents (S_1 and S_2) of two fish results in a nearly sinusoidal signal (S_1+S_2), whose amplitude, or envelope, is modulated at a rate equal to the difference in the frequencies of the two signals. For simplicity, the EODs are portrayed as sine wave signals. The signal frequency of fish no. 2 is assumed to be lower than that of no. 1, and as time progresses, the two signals alternately pass through periods of constructive and destructive interference, resulting in peaks and troughs in the envelope of the combined signal. The effect of EOD interference is shown for two points, A and B, on the body surface of fish no. 1. Electroreceptors only sense the current component oriented perpendicularly to the local body surface, and these components have been plotted in the traces underneath as simultaneous records for points A and B. Since the fish's own EOD current, indicated by solid arrows, has an internal source, it penetrates the body surface rather perpendicularly and at similar intensity at all points, and this condition also holds for the EOD substitute used in our experiments (see electrode E_s in figure 3.2). The neighbor's current (indicated by broken lines for two directions), however, hits the fish's surface at various angles. As a consequence, point A is more strongly affected by the neighbor's current than point B, and the combined signal, S_1+S_2, is therefore more strongly modulated in A than in B. The modulation in the combined signal's envelope is commonly referred to as a "beat pattern." For demonstration purposes, fewer cycles of the signal have been plotted per beat cycle than would be observed in a typical JAR situation. With the two fish having EOD frequencies of 400 and 404 Hz, respectively, the beat rate would be 4 Hz, and approximately 100 EOD cycles would be contained in one beat cycle. The diagram in (*b*) compares the signals perceived in A and B and shows that differences in the timing of their zero-crossings, or "phase," are modulated over the course of the beat cycle. In reference to the signal in B, the signal in A lags in phase while its amplitude falls and leads while its amplitude rises. This particular order in amplitude and phase modulations is due to the fact that the neighbor's EOD frequency is *lower* than the fish's own. If the neighbor's EOD frequency were higher, then a fall in the signal amplitude at A would be paired with a phase lead, and a rise in amplitude would be paired with a phase lag. Following the example in figure 2.2, the joint modulations in amplitude and phase can be recorded in a two-dimensional state plane, with the amplitude of the signal in A ($|S|_A$) plotted on the ordinate, and differential phase ($H_A–H_B$) plotted on the abscissa. In this case, since the EOD frequency of the neighbor is lower, a circular trajectory, or "graph," with a clockwise rotation is obtained if the more strongly modulated signal at A is evaluated in reference to the less strongly modulated signal at B. This two-dimensional presentation is shown in the diagram at the lower left, and the values of amplitude and phase have been plotted at a larger scale for clarity. A counterclockwise rotation would be obtained if the neighbor's signal frequency were higher. The sense of rotation thus reflects the sign of the Df between the neighbor's EOD and the fish's own. Much as the signal in A can be evaluated in reference to that in B, however, the signal in B can be evaluated symmetrically in reference to that in A (diagram at lower right). This graph is characterized by a smaller amplitude modulation, and, due to the inversion of the differential phase, its sense of rotation is opposite to that obtained for point A. (Note that the reciprocal evaluation of inputs from two points does not always produce graphs with opposite rotations but only if the vectors of the two interfering currents form similar angles, either acute or obtuse. If, by contrast, fish no. 1 compared inputs from A and from the opposite side of its body, then *both* graphs would rotate in the clockwise sense. This will be demonstrated later in figure 3.8)

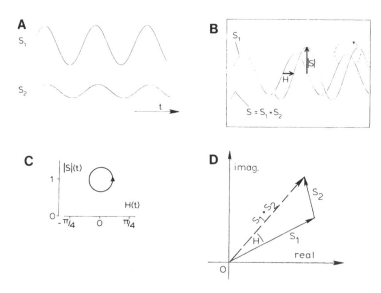

Figure 3.4
The interference of two sine wave signals with a Df generates modulations
in the amplitude and phase of the mixed signal, and the rate of modulation
is equal to the magnitude of Df. The modulations already portrayed in
figure 3.3 can conveniently be demonstrated with an oscilloscope and two
function generators. (A) Two sine wave signals plotted as functions of time
(t). The larger signal, S_1, represents the animal's own EOD; the smaller S_2
represents the EOD of a distant neighbor. (B) Schematic of an oscilloscope
display, triggered by the S_1 signal which, therefore, appears stationary. The
addition of S_1 and S_2 is shown on a separate beam to visualize the modu-
lations in amplitude ($|S|$) and phase (H) of the mixed signal in reference
to that of the pure S_1. With the frequency of S_2 being higher than that of
S_1, i.e., for a positive Df, the peak of the mixed signal is seen to rotate
about the stationary peak of S_1, Df times per second. The joint modulations
in amplitude and phase can be displayed in a two-dimensional plane (C) by
plotting successive pairs of $|S|$ and H values on the ordinate and abscissa,
respectively. As time progresses, these values generate a circular graph that
rotates counterclockwise for positive Dfs, and clockwise for negative Dfs,
at a rate equal to the magnitude of Df. The mean amplitude of the mixed
signal equals the amplitude of S_1, which is considered unity. A positive H
implies that the zero-crossing of the mixed signal lags with reference to
that of S_1. 2π corresponds to the period of the S_1 cycle, which is 2 ms long
if the frequency of S_1 is 500 Hz. (D) The values of $|S|$ and H can be calculated
by plotting S_1 and S_2 as complex vectors. The projections of the vectors of
S_1 and S_1+S_2 on the real axis then yield the functions of time plotted in
(B). S_1 is represented as a vector of unit length, rotating counterclockwise
around the origin, at its frequency f_1. The smaller vector S_2 is added to the

amplitude modulations in conjunction with the local phases measured in reference to an assumed pure representation of S_1, circular graphs are obtained that rotate at the same rate and in the counterclockwise direction if Df is positive (figure 3.5, center row). Due to the assumed larger contamination in A, modulations in amplitude and phase are larger in A than in B, and, consequently, the graph for A has a larger diameter than the graph for B. (Note also that a circular graph would collapse into a point as the relative amplitude of S_2 approached zero.) As the circles in A and B rotate in phase, they reach their peak amplitude positions in synchrony and always show phase values, H_A and H_B, of the same sign.

Since the animal has no absolute measure of phase, it could use phase differences between signals at two points of the body surface. It could, for example, extract phase information from A and B by "plotting" their differences rather then their individual values on the abscissae (figure 3.5, lower row). In this manner, an elliptical graph would be obtained for A which rotates counterclockwise and thus indicates a positive Df, whereas the elliptical graph obtained for B rotates clockwise and thus indicates a negative Df.

On the basis of this consideration, one could propose that areas A and B send opposite messages to the pacemaker to affect its firing frequency. Since the graph of area A is counterclockwise, it would cause the pacemaker to lower its frequency. Area B, having a clockwise graph, would induce a rise in the pacemaker frequency. Area A would win in this competition due to its larger amplitude modulation so that the animal would correctly lower its pacemaker

---

tip of S_1 and rotates at the rate Df around the tip of S_1, counterclockwise for positive Dfs and clockwise for negative Dfs. Therefore, S_2 rotates within the plane at the frequency $f_2 = f_1 + Df$ (note that Df is defined as $f_2 - f_1$). The length of the line connecting the origin with the end of $S_1 + S_2$ (broken line) represents the amplitude ($|S|$) of the mixed signal, whereas the angle between the broken line and S_1 represents its phase angle H. To agree with the presentation in (C), the value of H shown in this figure is considered negative to reflect a phase advance of the mixed signal. The maximal magnitude of H is obtained when S_2 forms a right angle with S_1, and, for relatively small S_2, this value is equal to the ratio (r) between the lengths of S_2 and S_1, measured in radians. The value of r corresponds to a temporal disparity, $\tau = r/(2\pi f_1)$, with $1/f_1$ being the period of S_1.

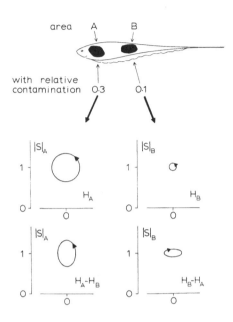

Figure 3.5
Eigenmannia has no absolute zero reference for computing phase information, but it obtains access to this information by computing differential
phase, i.e., the difference in pairs of phase values, H_A and H_B. Following
the demonstration in figure 3.3, assume that areas A and B are contaminated to different degrees by the interfering signal, S_2, so that modulation
graphs with different diameters are obtained for A and B (center row), with
$|S|_A$ and $|S|_B$ being local amplitudes and H_A and H_B being the corresponding
phases measured with reference to the phase of the uncontaminated S_1
cycle. With the frequency of S_2 being higher than that of S_1, i.e., Df being
positive, both graphs will circle counterclockwise. Further, as in figure 3.3,
assume that the spatial orientation of the S_2 field is such that the two
modulation graphs rotate in phase, i.e., reach their amplitude peaks in
synchrony and always have phase values of identical signs. As the animal
has no direct access to either H_A or H_B alone, but can extract their differences by comparing the timing of firing of local T-type receptors, it may
evaluate local amplitudes with reference to symmetrically calculated differential phases (bottom row). This operation yields an ellipse with counterclockwise rotation for A and an ellipse with clockwise rotation for B.
On the basis of the counterclockwise rotation in A, this area would inter-
pret the sign of Df as positive and 'vote' for a lowering of the pacemaker
frequency. An opposite vote would emerge from area B. Area A, however,
should win in this competition due to its larger amplitude modulation.
The arrows on the circles and ellipses mark an identical point in time.
(From Heiligenberg 1980)

frequency. If A and B were equally contaminated by S_2, as would occur under the condition of identical-geometry, H_A would equal H_B, and the graphs in the lower row of figure 3.5 would collapse into vertical lines and thus lack a sense of rotation. No JAR would then result from the interaction between A and B in this case, and this postulate is supported by the observation that JARs cannot be elicited under the identical-geometry condition, that is, when all areas of the body surface experience the same mixing ratio between the interfering signals.

A pandemonium of local computations and competing instructions

The proposal of competitive contributions from different areas of body surface can be tested experimentally by placing the animal into a two-compartment chamber with a tight silicone seal fitted around the animal's pectoral region, which provides sufficient electrical isolation between head and trunk (figure 3.6). Separate stimulus regimens can then be applied to these two portions of the animal's body. By placing one electrode in the animal's mouth and another one outside the fish within the same compartment, a sine wave stimulus can be applied to the head surface. Similarly, by placing one electrode, insulated up to its tip, into the dorsal musculature of the trunk and placing another electrode outside the fish within the same compartment, another sine wave stimulus can be applied to the rest of the body. A sine wave signal can be modulated electronically to simulate any form of amplitude and phase modulation independently (Heiligenberg and Bastian 1980). An identical sine wave carrier signal can thus be applied to head and trunk but modulated separately in each section to mimic the specific amplitude-phase graphs shown in the center row of figure 3.5, graph A for the head and graph B for the trunk. In this manner the whole surface of the head experiences graph A, while the whole surface of the trunk experiences graph B. As expected, the animal lowers its pacemaker frequency under this condition. If one now selectively increases only the amplitude modulation in B, without affecting its phase modulation, the animal's response vanishes gradually, as if a point of behavioral "titration" were reached. Moreover, a further

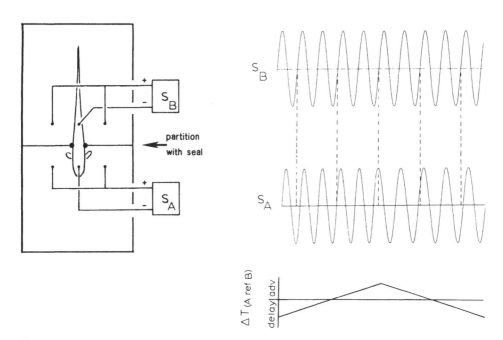

Figure 3.6
By placing a fish in a two-compartment chamber with a seal of high electrical resistance
fitted around its pectoral region, independent stimulus patterns (S_A and S_B) can be
applied to its head and trunk, respectively. For stimulating the head, one electrode is
placed inside the mouth, while two external, interconnected electrodes serve as references at a distance right and left from the animal. For stimulating the trunk, a
stainless steel needle, insulated except for its tip, is stuck into the dorsal musculature
to serve as an internal electrode. Due to the presence of internal electrodes, the current
vectors of each stimulus penetrate the body surface with the same polarity everywhere
in the compartment, much as shown for S_1 in figure 3.3. In a standard experiment, S_B
may be a pure sine wave, while S_A is a copy of this sine wave, modulated, for example,
in its phase (tracings at right). Specific differential phase values, or temporal disparities
(ΔT), generated by use of an analog delay line, can thus be imposed between the surface
of the head and the surface of the trunk. By using a sufficiently tight seal of silicone
grease, stimulus 'leakage' across the partition is not more than 1%.

increment of the amplitude in B induces a rise in the pacemaker frequency. Area B has won over area A at this point (Heiligenberg and Bastian 1980).

It should be noted at this point that, in order to achieve titration between head and trunk in this experiment, the amplitude modulation applied to the trunk must be larger than that applied to the head. If the amplitude modulations are equal in A and B, then the pacemaker frequency still falls. Due to a higher density of electroreceptors in the region of the head, electroreceptive fields on the head are more sensitive to amplitude modulations than receptive fields on the trunk, and this might explain why the representation of the head region carries more weight at a central level in its control of the JAR.

While the experiment described in figures 3.5 and 3.6 strongly supports the notion that the animal evaluates phase modulations in different areas of its body surface by a process equivalent to subtraction, such as $H_A–H_B$ in figure 3.5, another experiment directly confirms this assumption. By again using the two-compartment chamber paradigm of figure 3.6, an identical sine wave carrier is applied to head and trunk. While the carrier applied to the head is modulated in amplitude and phase to yield a circular graph rotating counterclockwise, the carrier applied to the trunk remains unmodulated, that is, its graph in the amplitude-phase plane is a point. Only the head, therefore, experiences an amplitude modulation, and the plot of this modulation in conjunction with the differential phase modulation between head and trunk yields a circular graph with counterclockwise rotation. As expected, this stimulus regimen causes the animal to lower its pacemaker frequency.

One may now switch the phase modulation functions between head and tail without affecting the amplitude modulation. For the head, this will result in a graph consisting of a point oscillating up and down on a vertical line (figure 3.7, lower row), while for the trunk, this will yield a point oscillating back and forth along a horizontal line. If the animal now "plotted" the amplitude modulation experienced by the head in conjunction with the differential phase modulation between head and trunk, a clockwise rotation should be obtained due to the inversion of the terms in the phase

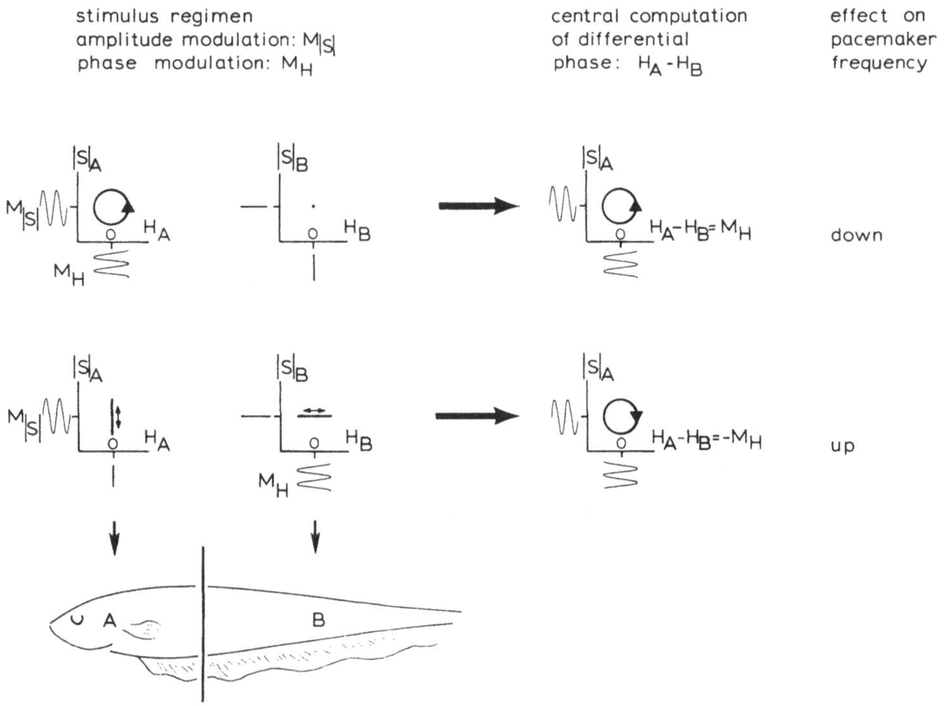

Figure 3.7
Eigenmannia evaluates differential phase by comparing the timing of zero-crossings of signals applied to different points on its body surface. In the experiment shown in the top row, a pure sine wave is applied to the trunk (as shown in figure 3.6), while a modulated version of this sine wave is applied to the head. Whereas the amplitude ($|S|_A$) is modulated by a sine function ($M_{|S|}$) the phase (H_A) is modulated by a cosine function (M_H). As a consequence, a circular graph with a counterclockwise rotation is obtained (upper left). Since the amplitude modulation at the head ($|S_A|$) plotted against the differential phase between head and trunk (H_A–H_B) yields a graph with a counterclockwise rotation, the animal lowers its pacemaker frequency. In the following experiment, the phase modulation functions applied to head and trunk are interchanged. This operation reverses the sense of rotation of the graph plotting $|S_A|$ versus H_A–H_B, and consequently, the animal reverses the shift of its pacemaker frequency. This experiment shows that the *difference* between phase values in the two regions is important and not the nature of the *local* modulation of phase.

function. As a consequence, the animal should raise its pacemaker frequency, and it does (Heiligenberg and Bastian 1980).

While the situation described in figures 3.3 and 3.5 points to a competitive interaction between two areas of body surface, figure 3.8 illustrates a case of synergism. Assume that the animal is exposed to a transverse S_2 field. As a consequence, the S_2 current will flow in the same direction as the S_1 current on one side of the body, while it will flow opposite to the S_1 current on the other side of the body (see figure 3.3). Maximal constructive interference on one side of the body will thus occur with maximal destructive interference on the opposite side. This means that a maximum in the beat envelope on the right side of the body will coincide with a minimum on the left side, and, as the two signals have different frequencies, this relation will reverse at a later point in the beat cycle, yielding a maximum on the left and a minimum on the right (figure 3.8). With regard to the beat cycle, the two sides of the body are out of phase by half a cycle. Yet a plot of the local amplitude modulation versus the differential phase modulation computed between the two sides of the body yields circular graphs with the same sense of rotation for both sides of the body. Both sides, therefore, should induce similar shifts in the pacemaker frequency. Figure 3.8 also shows that the differential phase measured between the two sides of the body is twice as large as that measured on either side in reference to an uncontaminated S_1, as it would be available on the fish's back or belly. Comparisons of inputs from body sites oriented opposite in reference to the current flow of a jamming signal thus should enhance the fish's ability to detect very small phase modulations.

Interactions between receptive fields on the body surface

The behavioral experiments reported in figures 3.5 to 3.7 convince us that the animal must evaluate amplitude modulations by reference to modulations in differential phase. At this point, one might already feel tempted to look into the neuronal implementations of these mechanisms. But even more details of this structure are provided by further behavioral experiments, which will be reviewed first.

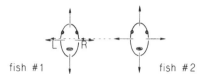

currents at point L

S_1

S_2

$S_1 + S_2$

currents at point R

S_1

S_2

$S_1 + S_2$

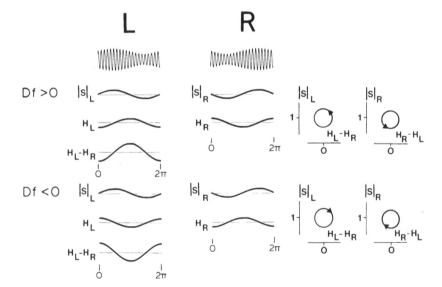

The two-compartment chamber introduced figure 3.6 allows us to present separate stimulus regimens to two sections of the animal's body surface to explore central mechanisms of their integration. Experiments performed in the multicompartment chamber shown in figure 3.9 provide additional insight. By presenting a sine wave signal, modulated in amplitude and phase, in any one compartment and providing an unmodulated signal as a phase reference in another compartment, one can demonstrate that the strongest JARs are obtained when the modulated signal is applied to the head, and progressively weaker JARs are elicited as the modulated signal is presented in more caudal compartments. Since switching of the phase modulations between compartments only reverses the sign

Figure 3.8
An external stimulus field (S_2) yields maximal modulations in the differential phase between sides of the body surface that experience opposite polarities of this stimulus. In the example shown in this figure, maximal modulations are obtained between the left and right sides of the body. The upper part of the figure, following the example of figure 3.3, shows currents recorded simultaneously on the left (L) and on the right (R), and in reference to the polarity of the local body surface. This implies that the S_2 current on the left is the negative version of that on the right. Since the fish's own signal (S_1; solid arrows), passes the two sides of the body with the same polarity in reference to the local body surfaces, while S_2 (broken arrows) passes the two sides with opposite polarities, the two currents will generate maximal destructive interference on one side whenever they generate maximal constructive interference on the opposite side. Therefore, the simultaneously recorded beat patterns, shown for the left and right side, are one half beat cycle out of phase. Their amplitudes, or beat envelopes, are labeled $|S|_L$ and $|S|_R$, respectively, and their phases, measured in reference to the phase of a pure S_1, are labeled H_L and H_R, respectively, with a phase lead plotted upwards. The mean value of $|S|$ is defined as unity, and the mean value of H is zero. For relatively small amplitudes of S_2, the modulations of amplitude and phase on one side are approximately negatives of those on the opposite side, i.e., $(|S|_L - 1) \approx -(|S|_R - 1)$ and $H_L \approx -H_R$. As a consequence, the differential phase, $H_L - H_R$ approximates $2H_L$, i.e., the differential phase measured between the two sides is twice as large as the phase measured in reference to the phase of a pure S_1. Most importantly, both sides experience the same sense of rotation in their respective amplitude-phase planes and thus cast identical votes for the control of the pacemaker frequency. This is in contrast to the situation depicted in figures 3.3 and 3.5, where comparisons between two areas yield opposite effects of different magnitudes.

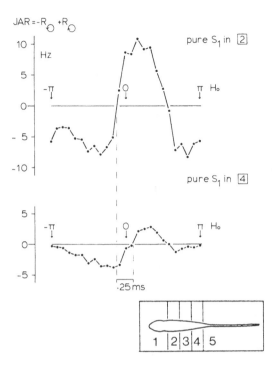

Figure 3.9
The spatial integration of sensory information can be studied in a multi-compartment chamber (inset at bottom), a modification of the two-compartment chamber shown in figure 3.6, with electrically tight seals fitted to every partition. In the graph at the top, a modulated sine wave signal is applied to the head compartment (1) and its unmodulated version, the "pure S_1," is applied as a reference to the second compartment. The mean phase of the signal at the head is offset by the value H_0 (abscissa) from the phase of the reference signal, and the JAR is measured, for every choice of H_0, as the mean difference between frequency shifts, R, caused by clockwise rotations and frequency shifts caused by counterclockwise rotations (ordinate). This graph shows that correct, i.e., *positive* JARs (see figure 3.2) are only obtained if H_0 is near zero (note that zero is the naturally occurring value). As the reference signal is applied to a more caudal compartment (lower graph), one can show that, with increasing spatial separation of the two stimuli, the JAR becomes weaker and incorrect frequency shifts are obtained for $H_0 = 0$. However, correct frequency shifts are obtained in this case if the signal applied to the head is appropriately delayed with reference to the signal applied caudally. The S_1 frequency in this experiment was 430 Hz, so that 2π is equivalent to 2.32 ms. The lower curve appears to be shifted to the right by 0.25 ms in reference to the upper curve. As will be shown later, this shift reflects conduction delays for afferent signals originating from more caudal receptors. The asymmetry of the upper graph with respect to $H_0 = 0$ reveals the relatively small delay between compartments 1 and 2. (From Heiligenberg and Bastian 1980)

of the frequency shifts but not their magnitude (see figure 3.7 and 3.11), the location of amplitude modulations on the body surface must determine the strength of the behavioral response. As was already suggested in connection with the experiments in figures 3.5 and 3.6, the higher density of P-type electroreceptors on the surface of the head appears to account for the higher sensitivity to amplitude modulations at the rostral end of the fish.

By increasing the distance between the two compartments receiving the stimuli, one obtains weaker JARs, and most importantly, the sign of the frequency shifts may reverse for sufficiently large distances (figure 3.9). However, the correct sign can be obtained by sufficiently advancing the mean phase of the more caudally applied stimulus (Heiligenberg and Bastian 1980). The attenuation of the JAR with increasing separation of the two receptive fields suggests that interactions between receptive fields in different parts of the body surface become weaker with increasing distance between them, and strong support for this assumption is found in the structural organization of a single lamina in the torus semicircularis where differential phase between receptive fields is computed (see chapter 4, The Torus Semicircularis). That the sign of frequency shifts is reversed with increasing distance between receptive fields can be explained on the basis of the experiments presented later in figures 3.11 and 3.12.

A line integration within the amplitude-phase plane

By independently modulating amplitude and phase of a sine wave carrier, one can generate patterns of modulations that a fish would never normally experience. Behavioral responses elicited by such unusual modulations tell us much about the central computational rules of the fish's perception, however. These experiments can be performed in the two-compartment chamber introduced in figure 3.6, with a pure sine wave signal applied to the trunk and its modulated version presented to the head. A variety of graphs can then be generated in the amplitude-phase plane by independent modulations of amplitude and phase. The normally occurring circular graphs can be replaced by squares, triangles, and loops of all kinds, and it is found that any graph that encloses an area in the clockwise sense raises the frequency of the pacemaker, while an enclosure in the counterclockwise sense of rotation lowers the frequency of the pacemaker (figure 3.10). Much as in the case of circular graphs, however, this only holds for graphs with a phase modulation centered near zero, and opposite frequency shifts are obtained as these graphs are shifted to mean phase values sufficiently far away from zero (figure 3.11) (Heiligenberg and Bastian 1980).

Besides presenting graphs as closed loops, one can present straight trajectories in the amplitude-phase plane, such as vertical or horizontal vectors. For example, in order to test the effect of a rise in amplitude at a given value of phase, one may increment the amplitude of the sine wave applied to the head over several successive carrier cycles, while keeping its phase constant in reference to the signal at the trunk. This form of modulation corresponds to a vector pointing upward in the amplitude-phase plane. The presentation of a single modulation cycle of this kind is insufficient to generate a noticeable shift in the fish's pacemaker frequency, and to present several such modulations in succession requires that one return to the starting point of the vector without generating additional contours in the amplitude-phase plane, which might affect the pacemaker frequency in their own way. The simplest solution to this problem appears to be a return to the beginning of the vector within a single carrier cycle. However, this jump represents a sudden drop in amplitude which, in spite of its short duration, is detected by higher-order neurons and, therefore, has its own behavioral consequences opposite to those of the gradual rise in amplitude (see chapter 4, The Electrosensory Lateral Line Lobe). Yet, as was pointed out previously, the strongest JARs are elicited by Dfs in the range of 2 to 6 Hz, and this rate of modulation can be translated into optimal increments or decrements in amplitude or phase per single carrier cycle. Vectors constructed with such increments represent gradual modulations that cause behavioral effects outweighing those of the sudden resetting. Nevertheless, the net frequency shifts obtained by such graphs are still small and are swamped by spontaneous frequency fluctuations in most individuals. Phase modulations alone have no significant effect upon the pacemaker

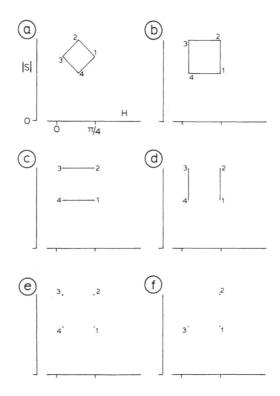

Figure 3.10
Artificial joint modulations of amplitude and phase that drive the JAR as
effectively as the naturally occurring circular graphs. Such graphs are generated by separate electronic modulations of the amplitude and phase of a
sine wave carrier signal presented in the head chamber, with the unmodulated carrier presented as a reference to a caudal chamber. Numbers
indicate the sequence of states, which is counterclockwise in all cases and,
accordingly, lowers the pacemaker frequency. For a carrier signal of 400
Hz, a modulation cycle covering 100 carrier cycles reflects a Df magnitude
of 4 Hz. While the graphs in (a) and (b) consist of gradual modulations
throughout, those in (c) and (d) contain jumps in either amplitude or phase.
The graphs in (e) and (f) contain jumps in amplitude and phase; each point
in the graph is maintained for an equal number of carrier cycles. (From
Heiligenberg and Bastian 1980)

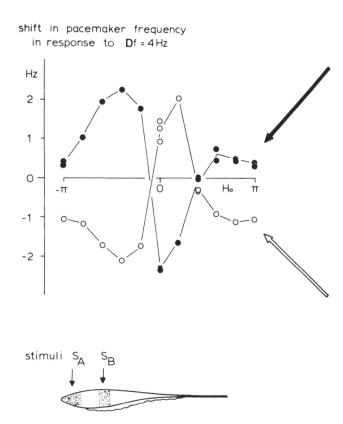

Figure 3.11
Correct JARs are only obtained if modulation graphs have mean phase values (H_0) in the vicinity of zero. (But also note the effect of a wider spatial separation of stimuli shown in figure 3.9). A signal (S_A) applied to the head, is modulated in amplitude and phase to yield a counterclockwise rotation, with a mean phase (H_0) in reference to the phase of the unmodulated signal (S_B) applied to the trunk. The counterclockwise rotation, which reflects a positive Df, should lower the pacemaker frequency. This effect, however, is only observed for H_0 values near zero (filled circles). As was demonstrated in figure 3.7, all frequency shifts are reversed if the phase modulations of the two stimuli, S_A and S_B, are interchanged (open circles). The variables marked by asterisks represent the modulation functions used in each experiments. Scaling factors and offsets are left out for simplicity. The computation in the lower right shows that switching of the phase modulations between head and trunk is mathematically equivalent to a reversal of the sign of Df. The effects demonstrated in this figure for circular modulations are also observed if unnatural modulation graphs as shown in figure 3.10 are used instead. (From Heiligenberg 1980).

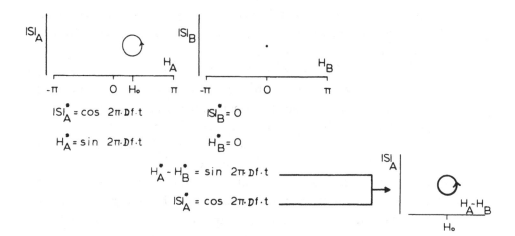

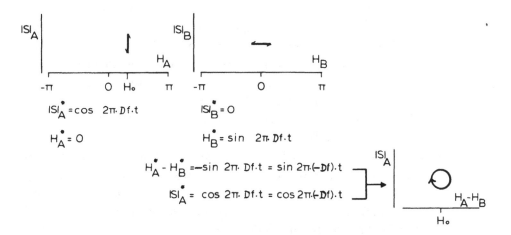

frequency, while amplitude rises and falls change the pacemaker frequency as a function of their associated phase value (Heiligenberg and Bastian 1980) (figure 3.12)

As illustrated in figure 3.12, the effect of a closed graph in the amplitude-phase plane can be formulated as a line integral taken along its contour. Amplitude modulations executed within specific phase ranges to the right and to the left of zero have stronger effects than those associated with larger or smaller absolute phase values, and this explains why a circle centered at phase zero causes a frequency shift opposite to that of the same circle centered sufficiently far away from phase zero. As will be shown in chapter 4 (The Gating of Amplitude Information by Phase Information), action potentials generated by T-receptors distant to the brain arrive later in the central nervous system than those generated by proximal T-receptors. As a consequence, the neuronal representations of graphs resulting from the phase comparisons between proximal and distal receptive fields are no longer centered at phase zero and, therefore, cause incorrect frequency shifts of the pacemaker. One can, however, compensate for this physiological limitation by appropriately delaying the phase of the stimulus applied to the head with reference to that of the stimulus applied to the more distant area on the trunk (see figure 3.9, lower graph).

Figure 3.12 already suggests that the effects of amplitude modulations may be gated by the associated state of differential phase, and this assumption will be supported by physiological evidence in chapter 4. There, it will also be shown that neurons discriminating the differential phase between two points on the body surface respond most strongly within phase ranges that roughly correspond to those that are also most effective in the behavioral tests described in figure 3.12.

Jamming by multiple stimuli and higher harmonics

The validity of the line integral algorithm presented in figure 3.12 can be tested by presenting the more complicated patterns of modulation that result from the interference of more than two EODs. If the animal's EOD, or S_1, is jammed by the signals, S_2 and S_3, of two neighbors, modulation graphs are obtained whose shape and

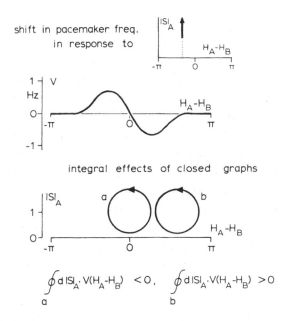

Figure 3.12
The effect of a closed graph can be interpreted as the integral of contributions from line segments that constitute this graph. Vertical streaks, representing amplitude modulations, are most significant, and their effect depends upon the associated phase value, H. A fish is placed in a two-compartment chamber as shown in figure 3.6, with a pure sine wave signal, S_B, applied to the trunk and a modulated version of this signal applied as S_A to the head. The form of modulation is shown in the inset in the upper right: A gradual increase in the amplitude $(|S|_A)$ executed at a fixed differential phase $(H_A–H_B)$. The upper diagram shows the shift (V) of the pacemaker frequency induced by this form of modulation as a function of the differential phase. The negative of this function is obtained if $|S|_A$ is decremented rather than incremented. The scale of this function varies considerably among individuals, and for most the behavioral data are so noisy that the general shape of this function can hardly be recognized. The lower diagram shows how the effect of a closed graph can be computed as a line integral. As indicated by the notation underneath, incremental, vertical displacements $(d|S|_A)$ along the circle must be multiplied by the local value of the V-function, and these products are to be summed over the whole path of the circle, with incremental upward displacements counting positively and incremental downward displacements counting negatively. As a consequence of this algorithm, a circle with a counterclockwise rotation should lower the pacemaker frequency if centered at phase zero (a) but raise the pacemaker frequency if centered away from phase zero (b). This is observed in behavioral experiments as shown in figure 3.11. (From Heiligenberg 1980)

periodicity depend on the relative intensities of these two signals as well as on their respective Dfs relative to the frequency of S_1. The resulting trajectories in the amplitude-phase plane can be quite complex in this electric fish version of the three-body problem (figure 3.13). By adding S_2 and S_3 electronically and presenting this mixed signal, instead of a single S_2 as in the previously described experiments, shifts in pacemaker frequency can be induced which can be predicted by line integration of the respective graphs (Partridge and Heiligenberg 1980). Problems arise for the multiple-looped graphs shown in the center of the lower row of figure 3.13, however. These particular graphs, being composed of very similar Dfs of opposite signs, require 5 s for the completion of a full cycle, and this period appears to be longer than the internal integration time of the animal. This issue will be addressed again in chapter 4.

The representation of stimulus patterns as graphs in a two-dimensional plane also offers an explanation for earlier findings by Bullock et al. (1972). These authors reported that *Eigenmannia* shows a JAR in response to a jamming stimulus whose frequency differs by a small amount, Df, from a higher harmonic of the fish's fundamental EOD frequency, but that no JAR can be elicited by stimulating the fish with frequencies near subharmonics of its EOD. Most significantly, these authors reported that the optimal magnitudes of Df were the same, between 2 and 6 Hz, for stimulating the fish near its fundamental or near its higher harmonics. Although the fish's natural EOD does contain higher harmonics, this result does not depend on their presence, as replacement of the EOD by a pure sine wave does not affect these responses (Heiligenberg et al. 1978b). This result can readily be interpreted by analyzing the corresponding modulation graphs. Following the procedures outlined in figure 3.4D, the amplitude ($|S|$) and phase (H) of the interference signal can be calculated by presentation of the fish's own signal (S_1) and the interfering signal (S_2) as vectors rotating in the complex plane. If $|S|$ and H are then plotted in a two-dimensional plane, continuous graphs are obtained if the frequency of S_2 is close to a higher harmonic of S_1, and these graphs repeat themselves at a rate that is equal to the magnitude of the Df with respect to the nearest harmonic frequency of S_1. When the frequency of S_2 is close to a

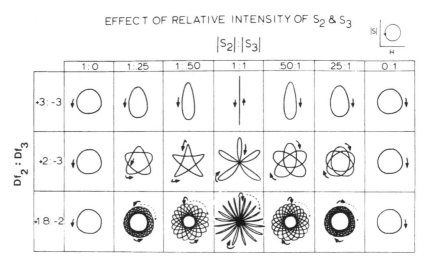

Figure 3.13
The interference of two signals (S_2 and S_3) with the fish's own (S_1) generates modulations in the amplitude-phase plane that depend on the relative amplitudes of the two interfering signals as well as on their respective frequency differences (Df_2 and Df_3) with respect to S_1. These graphs can be constructed by plotting the three signals as vectors rotating in the complex plane so that S is the vector sum $S_1 + S_2 + S_3$, |S| is the length of S, and H is the phase angle between S and S_1 (see figure 3.4D). The maximal magnitude of either S_2 or S_3, indicated by the value 1 in the top line, is 20% that of S_1. Solid vectors indicate the motion along the contours of the graph, broken vectors indicate the direction in which loops of more complex graphs are formed over time. (From Partridge and Heiligenberg 1980)

subharmonic of S_1, however, isolated points are obtained which jump back and forth across the plane so that a tracing of their temporal sequence forms a starburst pattern (figure 3.14). This demonstrates that the JAR requires stimulus patterns that yield consistent progressions within the phase-amplitude plane and that such patterns are most effective if they repeat themselves at a rate between 2 and 6 Hz. Note that such progression need not be gradual and continuous throughout. Discontinuities as shown in the graphs of figure 3.10 *c-f*, do not impair the performance of the JAR as long as a sufficient number of consecutive EOD cycles share similar phase and amplitude values. This observation can readily be explained on the basis of the response properties of receptors and higher-order neurons described in chapter 4.

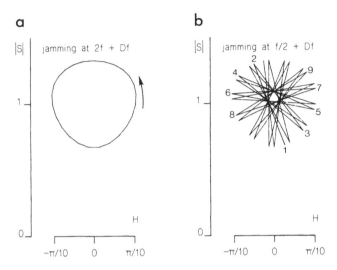

Figure 3.14
(a) The interference of the fish's EOD with a weaker signal of a frequency
near the second harmonic of the EOD generates a smooth modulation in
the amplitude (|S|) and phase (H) of the mixed signal. Amplitude and phase
of the mixed signal were calculated by representing the EOD and the
interfering signal as pure sine waves, S_1 and S_2, rotating as vectors in the
complex plane (see figure 3.4D). The frequency (f_1) of S_1 is 100 Hz, and the
frequency (f_2) of S_2 is *twice* the frequency of S_1 plus a positive Df of 4 Hz,
i.e., $f_2 = 204$ Hz. The amplitude of S_2 is one third that of S_1. This graph
consists of $f_1/Df = 100/4 = 25$ points that have been connected by straight
lines in their temporal sequence. This graph rotates counterclockwise and
repeats itself four (=Df) times per second. The same graph would be
obtained if the frequency of S_2 differed by the same Df from the *fundamental* frequency of S_1, i.e., if f_2 were 104 Hz instead of 204 Hz. (b) The
interference of the fish's EOD with a weaker signal of a frequency near the
first subharmonic of the EOD generates isolated and distantly spaced points
in the amplitude-phase plane. Same values, calculation and presentation
as in (a), with the exception that f_2 is 54 Hz ($f_2 = \frac{1}{2}f_1 + Df$) rather than
204 Hz. The points of this graph lie at the periphery and are connected in
their temporal order by straight lines. Since sequential points lie on opposite sides of the circle, their connection by straight lines forms a starburst
pattern. The first nine points are labeled.

4 Neuronal Implementation of the Jamming Avoidance Response

This presentation will start at the receptor level and follow the flow of information to the generation of the behavioral response. It is our goal to explain all behavioral phenomena of the jamming avoidance response (JAR) on the basis of specific properties of its neuronal implementation. In general, we want to learn how networks of neurons extract behaviorally relevant stimulus patterns and convert this information for the control of behavioral responses. We will explore whether the recognition of specific stimulus patterns depends on the activation of individual "recognition" neurons or on the distributed activation of large populations of neurons with more general response properties. We will also ask to what extent extraordinary perceptual acuities revealed at the behavioral level can be traced to the performance of individual neurons. The description of this research will further show how behavioral experiments inspire physiological studies, and how discoveries made at the single-cell level suggest tests of potentially related behavioral phenomena. Most importantly, however, it will become apparent that the representation of JAR-related stimulus patterns within the amplitude-phase plane is not only very effective with regard to its analytical and predictive power but also matches the structural and functional organization of the neuronal hardware of the JAR.

A general outline of the electrosensory pathways through the fish's brain was given in figure 3.1. Electroreceptors are present on the fish's body surface and project, via primary afferents, to four somatotopically ordered maps in the bilateral electrosensory lateral line lobe (ELL) of the hindbrain (figure 4.1). The maps of the ELL, in turn, project topographically to a single map in the multilayered torus semicircularis of the midbrain. The torus, which is homolo-

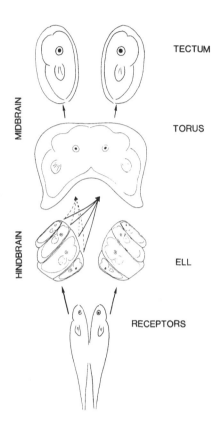

Figure 4.1
The spatial order of electrosensory information is preserved in layers of
higher-order neurons in the hindbrain and midbrain due to their somatotopic organization. Electroreceptors on the fish's body surface project ipsi-
laterally, via primary afferents, to four somatotopically ordered maps in the
ELL of the hindbrain. Whereas ampullary receptors project only to the most
medial map, each tuberous receptor projects to the three remaining maps
via collaterals of its primary afferent. The maps of the ELL project predominantly to the contralateral side of a single, multilayered map in the torus
semicircularis of the midbrain. An ipsilateral topographic projection of the
torus to the tectum leads to a convergence of visual and electrosensory
spatial information.

gous to the inferior colliculus of mammals, projects topographically to the tectum, which is homologous to the superior colliculus of mammals. The projections of primary afferents to the ELL are ipsilateral, the projections to the torus are predominantly contralateral, and the projections from torus to tectum are again ipsilateral. Therefore, the electrosensory surface of the right half of the body maps onto the left tectum. Since the tectum also receives a retinotopic projection from the contralateral eye, visual and electrosensory information can be brought into spatial register to yield a multimodal map of the environment (Bastian 1982). The tectum contains the highest known level of spatially ordered electrosensory information and also shows a topographically ordered representation of the direction of intended swimming (Yuthas 1985). Still higher-level structures, such as the nucleus electrosensorius and the prepacemaker nucleus of the diencephalon, contain premotor stations for the control of different frequency modulations of the pacemaker.

The following sections begin at the receptor periphery and follow the flow of information to higher levels of the nervous system.

THE CODING OF AMPLITUDE AND PHASE MODULATIONS BY TUBEROUS ELECTRORECEPTORS

Gymnotiform fish have two types of tuberous electroreceptors, P-type and T-type, which are well suited for the coding of amplitude and phase modulations in EOD-like signals (Scheich et al. 1973). The somata of their primary afferents are located in the anterior lateral line nerve ganglion. Action potentials of primary afferents can be recorded either within this ganglion or in the branches of lateral line nerves leading to this ganglion. Afferents from P-type receptors, commonly referred to as *P-units*, fire intermittently and increase their rate of firing with a rise in stimulus amplitude. *T-units* fire one spike on each cycle of the stimulus, phase-locked with little jitter to the zero-crossing of the signal (figure 4.2).

While presenting a periodic pattern of amplitude and phase modulations to an immobilized fish, one may monitor the activity of various P-units and T-units and store these records together with a

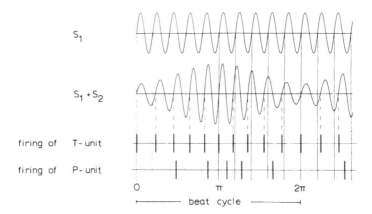

Figure 4.2
The coding of modulations in instantaneous phase and amplitude by T-type and P-type tuberous electroreceptors, a schematic representation. The trace at the top represents the fish's EOD signal (S_1). The second trace shows the interference pattern resulting from addition of a neighbor's signal (S_2). This beat pattern is characterized by a modulation of the instantaneous amplitude, or envelope, of the signal and by a modulation of its instantaneous phase, or the timing of its zero-crossings (marked by broken lines), in reference to that of the pure S_1 (marked by continuous lines). The two traces at the bottom indicate the coding of the phase and amplitude modulations by T-unit and P-unit afferents. The phase of the signal is coded by the timing of a single action potential fired by T-unit afferents within each S_1 cycle and at a fixed latency with reference to the timing of the positive zero-crossing. The difference in the timing of action potentials of T-units in different parts of the body surface would thus reflect the differential phase between the respective signals. The modulations in the amplitude of the signal are coded by a corresponding modulation in the probability of P-unit afferents firing an action potential within the current S_1 cycle.

marker that indicates the beginning of each modulation cycle. By means of this marker, one can then align the activity records of a P-unit and of a T-unit with reference to the modulation cycle and plot these two records in a two-dimensional plane to portray their joint responses to this particular modulation pattern. The top row of figure 4.3 shows the amplitude and phase modulations that would result from the interference with a neighbor's EOD whose frequency is higher than that of the animal's own EOD. The bottom row of this figure displays the corresponding responses of a P-unit and of

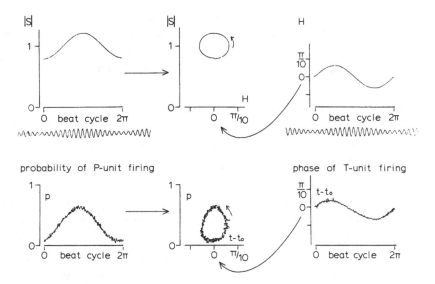

Figure 4.3
Patterns of phase and amplitude modulations are coded by the joint activation of T-units and P-units. Top row: A beat cycle, generated by the
interference of the fish's own signal (S₁) with that of a neighbor (S₂) is
characterized by a modulation of the instantaneous amplitude (|S|; far left),
and by a modulation of the instantaneous phase (H; far right). A plot of |S|
versus H in a two-dimensional plane (center) yields a circular graph that
rotates counterclockwise for positive Dfs, i.e., when the frequency of S₂ is
higher than that of S₁. Bottom row: The modulation in amplitude is coded
by the probability (p) of P-unit firing, while the modulation in phase is
coded by the timing (t) of T-unit firing, measured in reference to the timing
(t₀) of T-unit firing in an area less strongly contaminated by S₂. A plot of p
versus t–t₀ yields a circular graph that preserves the sense of rotation of
the corresponding graph in the |S|,H plane. The data for p and t–t₀ in the
lower row are mean values obtained from data collected over 25 beat cycles.
The beat cycle covers a fixed number of S₁ cycles, and the value of p, for a
given cycle of S₁ within the beat cycle, is measured by the mean number
of spikes obtained within that particular S₁ cycle. The value of t is the
mean spike latency at a given S₁ cycle, measured in reference to its start.
For negative Dfs, the values of H and t–t₀ would be the negatives of those
shown in this figure, while the associated records of |S| and p would be
identical. As a consequence, the circular graphs in the center would rotate
in the clockwise direction. (From Heiligenberg and Partridge 1981)

a T-unit. The diagram in the center of this figure shows that the counterclockwise rotation in the amplitude-phase plane maps onto a counterclockwise rotation in a two-dimensional plane portraying the joint activities of the P-unit and of the T-unit.

Behavioral consequences of receptor dynamics

The joint activity of P-units and T-units even reproduces the more complex graphs generated by the interference of two jamming signals with the animal's EOD. Here, certain distortions become more evident, however (figure 4.4).

The discharge rate of a P-unit increases with the steady-state amplitude of a stimulus as well as with the temporal derivative of the amplitude. Therefore, the firing rate not only codes the current amplitude level but also shows transient rises and falls in response to sudden increments and decrements in stimulus amplitude, respectively. As a consequence, the firing rate of a P-unit briefly overshoots a steep rise in stimulus amplitude and undershoots a sudden drop. This property not only distorts the symmetry of the respective graphs in the two-dimensional plane (compare the responses to clockwise and counterclockwise rotations in figure 4.4) but may also introduce small additional loops (see triangular graph in figure 4.4).

The pattern of P- and T-unit activity in response to an even more detailed graph, such as the "flower" in figure 4.5, bears little resemblance to the graph in the amplitude-phase plane, unless one inspects individual sections of the pattern. Although every petal in this graph has a counterclockwise sense of rotation, some of their receptor-coded representations show the opposite rotation. This means that the animal perceives a sequence of clockwise rotations followed by a sequence of counterclockwise rotations, and this process will repeat itself as the joint modulation in amplitude and phase progresses through successive petals of the flower pattern. With one jamming stimulus of this pattern being 1.0 Hz higher than the animal's EOD substitute, and the other jamming stimulus being 0.9 Hz lower, the whole graph repeats itself every 10 s, and as a graph of this kind cycles so slowly in the amplitude-phase

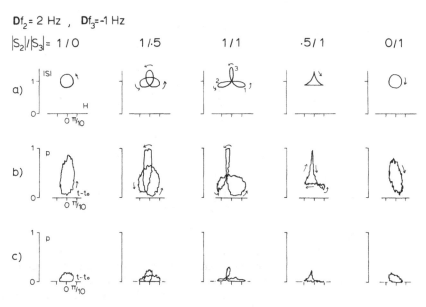

Figure 4.4
P-unit and T-unit afferents also code the more complicated graphs generated by the interference of two signals (S₂ and S₃) with the fish's own signal (S₁). The shape of these graphs (top row) depends on the relative amplitudes of S₂ and S₃ as well as on their respective Dfs with reference to the frequency of S₁. At the |S₂|/|S₃| ratio of 1/1 (center), the two stimuli are equally strong, with each having one-third of the amplitude of S₁. The ensuing graph with three loops follows the course indicated by arrows and repeats itself once per second (due to Df₃ = −1 Hz). The graphs to the left and right have increasingly weaker amplitudes of S₃ and S₂, respectively, and turn into circles with directions and rates of rotation associated with the sole presence of S₂ or S₃. Rows (b) and (c) show data from two different sets of neurons responding to the graphs in the top row. These data were obtained as outlined in figure 4.3. The lower overall probability of firing of the P-unit in row (c) causes the corresponding neuronal graphs to be compressed vertically. The less distorted representations in row (b) show minor deviations from the ideal shapes shown in the top row. These deviations occur because the firing of P-units not only reflects the current level of signal amplitude but to some extent also follows its temporal derivative. (From Heiligenberg and Partridge 1981)

$$Df_2 = 1\,Hz \ , \quad Df_3 = -0.9\,Hz \ , \quad |S_2|/|S_3| = 1/1$$

a)   b)

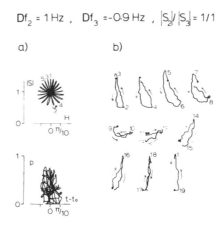

Figure 4.5
By choosing two jamming signals (S_2 and S_3) with Dfs of opposite signs and a smaller difference in magnitudes than in the case of the center graph in figure 4.4, graphs with a larger number of loops are obtained (top figure in a). The loops of this graph are generated in the sequence indicated by the numbers, with each loop being traced in the counterclockwise direction. The whole graph requires 10 s to be traversed. The neuronal representation of this graph appears scrambled when plotted in its entirety (lower graph in a). A plot of the representation of individual loops in (b), with numbers and arrows referencing corresponding sections in (a), reveals that some show a correct, counterclockwise trace, while others show an incorrect, clockwise trace. This distortion in the neuronal representation is due to the dynamics of P-unit responses (see legend to figure 4.4). The behavioral consequences of this distortion are shown in figure 4.6. (From Heiligenberg and Partridge 1981)

plane, one can indeed observe that the pacemaker frequency gently rises and falls (figure 4.6) as the animal successively experiences clockwise and counterclockwise representations of individual petals. These distortions in the neuronal code of this stimulus pattern thus lead to behavioral responses that can be predicted on the basis of the line-integral algorithm introduced in connection with figure 3.12.

Further support for this theory is provided by experiments with jamming frequencies in the vicinity of higher and lower harmonics of the fish's EOD. As stated in connection with figure 3.14, JARs can also be elicited by jamming stimuli of a frequency near a higher

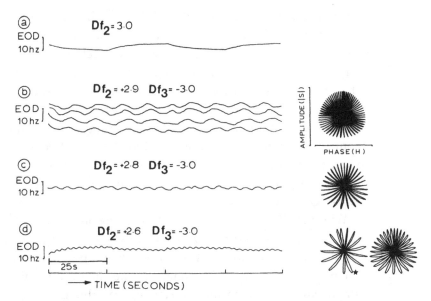

Figure 4.6
JARs to a single interfering stimulus (*a*) and to a pair of such stimuli with difference frequencies (Df$_2$ and Df$_3$) of similar magnitudes but opposite signs (*b-d*). Shifts in EOD frequency are plotted on the ordinates. (*a*) A single jamming signal (S$_2$) is applied at a frequency that initially is maintained 3 Hz higher than that of the fish's EOD, i.e., Df$_2$ = +3 Hz. The sign of Df$_2$ is then switched every 25 s, causing the fish to alternately lower and raise its EOD frequency in a futile attempt to increase the magnitude of the frequency difference between the jamming signal and its own EOD. (*b*) An addition of two jamming signals (S$_2$ and S$_3$) of equal amplitudes is applied with Df$_2$ and Df$_3$ initially being +2.9 and −3.0 Hz, respectively. Every 25 s, the signs of the Dfs are reversed. Since the magnitudes of the two Dfs differ so little, there is no net shift of the EOD frequency over any 25 s interval. However, the stimulus modulation graph shown on the right repeats itself every 10 s and causes modulations in the EOD frequency with a period of the same length. As outlined in figure 4.5, these modulations can be explained in that the neuronal representations of the loops of the modulation graph go through sequences of clockwise and counterclockwise tracings and thus alternately cause rises and falls of the EOD frequency. (*c*) same as (*b*), but with Df$_2$ = +2.8 Hz instead. The corresponding graph repeats itself every 5 s, and modulations with the same periodicity are seen in the EOD record. (*d*) same as (*b*), but with Df$_2$ = +2.6 Hz. The corresponding graph repeats itself entirely every 5 s, but the individual loops perform two full rotations over this period of time (the first round is shown in the left inset, the full graph is shown in the right inset). The graph thus has a periodicity of 2.5 s, and modulations at the same periodicity are seen in the EOD record. (From Partridge and Heiligenberg 1980)

harmonic of the animal's EOD, while stimuli of a frequency near a subharmonic fail to elicit JARs (Bullock et al. 1972). As one records the activity of P- and T-units exposed to such jamming regimens, one can, by following the example of figure 4.3, generate graphs that plot the modulation of the probability (p) of P-unit firing and the modulation of the differential timing $(t-t_0)$ of T-unit firing in a two-dimensional plane. As illustrated in figure 3.14, smooth and continuous graphs are only obtained for jamming frequencies in the vicinity of a higher harmonic (figure 4.7), whereas graphs obtained in the case of subharmonics are discontinuous (Heiligenberg and Partridge 1981).

While all T-units show very similar responses under such jamming conditions, P-units vary individually in their responses to amplitude modulations. As a consequence, the shape of a graph in the $p/(t-t_0)$ plane depends strongly on the choice of P-unit. Circular graphs are obtained in most instances, and the majority of P-units also yields the correct sense of rotation (six cases on the left in figure 4.7). However, some P-units yield figure-eight patterns that contain both directions of rotation. These figure-eights resemble graphs that are obtained if one plots the actual beat envelope versus the timing of zero-crossings (figure 4.7a, right), rather than the mathematically defined amplitude ($|S|$) versus the phase (H). At this point, it is not clear which choice of variables portrays the response properties of tuberous electroreceptors most accurately. Yet, that most receptors generate graphs with the correct sense of rotation can explain why *Eigenmannia* correctly recognizes the sign of the frequency difference (Df) if jamming stimuli have frequencies near higher harmonics of its EOD.

Effects of harmonic distortions in EOD substitutes

Finally, the analysis of receptor responses to EOD-like signals has solved an earlier theoretical controversy about the mechanism of the JAR. After Scheich and Bullock (1974) and Scheich (1977) had discovered that JARs could be elicited in a curarized fish by substituting an EOD mimic for its silenced EOD, they reported that JARs could only be evoked after the sinusoidal EOD mimic had been clipped in one polarity to resemble the natural EOD waveform. More specifically, they reported that correct JARs could only be elicited if the polarity of the clipped EOD mimic corresponded to that of the natural EOD and that wrong frequency shifts were obtained after the polarity of the EOD mimic had been inverted. However, later experiments by Heiligenberg et al. (1978b) revealed that pure sine waves were sufficient EOD substitutes for eliciting JARs as long as the EOD mimic and the jamming signal were offered through different sets of electrodes to ensure differential contamination of the EOD mimic by the jamming stimulus over the animal's body surface. Yet, if the EOD mimic and the jamming stimulus were added electronically and then presented through the same pair of electrodes, JARs could no longer be elicited unless the EOD mimic was clipped as in the original experiments by Scheich and Bullock. The JAR-like frequency shifts elicited in the latter case were found to be very small compared to those obtained when the EOD mimic and the jamming stimulus were offered through separate sets of electrodes, however. Moreover, all animals indeed reversed the direction of their frequency shifts with a reversal of the polarity of the clipped EOD mimic. But while some individuals behaved in accordance with the original claim by shifting in the correct direction if the polarity of the EOD mimic corresponded to that of the natural EOD waveform, other individuals did exactly the opposite. What was even more revealing was that an animal might produce the "correct" behavior for several minutes and then slowly, after minutes of small and unpredictable frequency fluctuations, switch to "incorrect" behavior. It was apparent from these observations that the animals had no unambiguous cue about the sign of the frequency difference, Df, as long as the EOD mimic and the jamming signal were offered through the same pair of electrodes. Why then did they shift their frequency at all if the EOD mimic was clipped? An answer is found by studying responses of electroreceptors under these conditions.

If the EOD mimic and the jamming stimulus are added electronically and presented through the same pair of electrodes, then all of the body surface will experience the same mixing ratio between

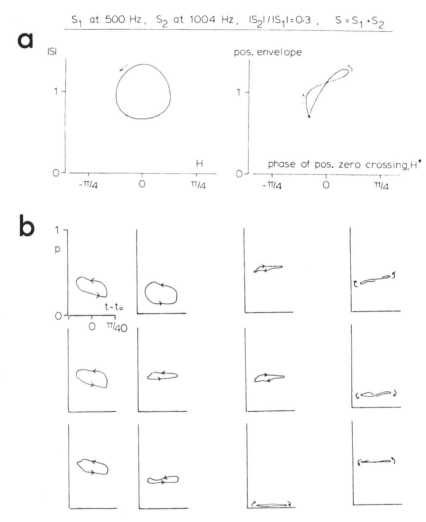

Figure 4.7
The interference of the fish's EOD signal (S_1) with a jamming signal, S_2, at a frequency near the fish's second harmonic causes smooth and continuous modulations in the amplitude-phase plane and similar modulations in the neuronal representations. a) The graph on the left is a plot of signal amplitude ($|S|$) versus phase (H) as calculated from the representation of S_1 and S_2 as vectors in the complex plane (see figure 3.14). The graph on the right is a plot of the positive envelope of the interference pattern versus the timing of actual zero-crossings of the signal. These two variables were obtained from a numerical simulation of the wave form ($S_1 + S_2$). (Note that the positive envelope would be identical to $|S|$, and the timing of zero-crossings

these two signals, and, consequently, no modulation in the differential phase between any two sites should occur. This particular condition is referred to as the *identical-geometry condition* (see figure 3.3), and it implies that the graphs in the amplitude-phase plane collapse into vertical streaks, which lack a sense of rotation and therefore offer no clue about the sign of Df. Is this also true for the corresponding graphs portraying the joint P-unit and T-unit activity under the identical-geometry condition?

By recording a number of P-units and T-units for positive and negative values of Df, one can, following the example in figure 4.3, generate graphs of their joint activity by plotting the firing rate of one P-unit on the ordinate and plotting the difference in the timing of the spikes of two chosen T-units on the abscissa. As originally reported by Bullock and Chichibu (1965), some T-units are somewhat sensitive to amplitude modulations and advance the timing of their action potentials with increasing stimulus amplitude. By choosing one T-unit of this kind and another T-unit that is insensitive to amplitude modulations, the difference in the timing of their spikes is then seen to be modulated during the beat cycle and to reach a maximum at the peak of the stimulus amplitude. But even with this choice of two T-units, the resulting graphs fail to open and are identical streaks for positive and negative Dfs as long as the two interfering signals are pure sine waves (see example in figure 4.8a,b). Therefore, the animal can extract no information

---

would be identical to H if the frequency of S_2 were in the vicinity of the frequency of S_1, rather than in the vicinity of a frequency twice as high.) Both graphs are generated 4 times per second, in accordance with Df = 4 Hz (Df = 1004 Hz − 1000 Hz, with 1000 being the first harmonic above 500). In agreement with the positive sign of Df, the graph on the left follows a counterclockwise rotation, and the fish lowers its pacemaker frequency. Responses of 12 different P-units to this stimulus pattern are shown in (b). In each diagram, the probability (p) of firing of a P-unit has been plotted against the differential timing (t−t₀) of the firing of one and the same T-unit (same presentation as in figure 4.3). The six P-units portrayed on the left yield graphs with the correct sense of rotation. The three P-units in the center yield flat graphs with the incorrect rotation. Finally, the three P-units at the right yield figure-eight graphs similar to the graph on the right in (a). (From Heiligenberg and Partridge 1981)

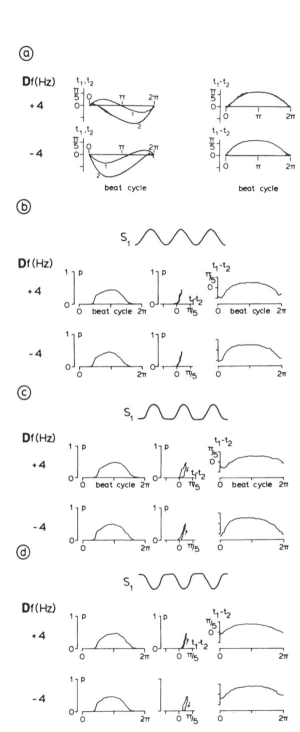

about the sign of Df under this condition and, accordingly, shows no JAR.

If the sine wave mimicking the EOD is now clipped in one polarity (figure 4.8c), the same set of neurons generates graphs that open up to form loops and reveal opposite senses of rotation for positive and negative Dfs. If the polarity of the EOD mimic is then reversed (figure 4.8d), the same graphs reverse their senses of rotation for each sign of Df. This observation readily explains why clipped EOD mimics can induce JAR-like shifts under the identical-geometry condition, and why the frequency shifts of the pacemaker reverse their directions with a reversal of the polarity of the EOD mimic.

Figure 4.8
Clipping of a sinusoidal EOD substitute (S_1) may provide ambiguous cues about the sign of the frequency difference (Df) between a jamming signal and the fish's own signal. In all experiments described in this figure, a sinusoidal jamming signal (S_2) was added electronically to the EOD substitute (S_1) and then presented through the same pair of electrodes, one electrode in the fish's mouth and one at the tip of its tail. As a consequence, all points on the body surface experienced the same mixture of the two signals. The amplitude of S_2 was one-third of that of S_1. (a) Left: Phases t_1 and t_2 of the firing of two T-units during beat cycles with positive and negative Dfs. The maximum of the beat envelope is at π. In contrast to unit 1, unit 2 advances its phase of firing with an increase of the amplitude of the signal. Consequently, its phase advance is maximal near the center of the beat cycle where the amplitude ($|S|$) of the combined signal (S_1+S_2) is maximal. Many intermediates are found between the amplitude-insensitive unit 1 and the highly sensitive unit 2. Right: Difference in timing, or differential phase (t_1-t_2), of T-unit firing for positive and negative Dfs. (b–d) Responses of one P-unit and two T-units tested under three different S_1 regimens (see insets at top): a pure sine wave (b), a sine wave clipped in the negative polarity (c), and a sine wave clipped in the positive polarity (d). The amplitude of S_1 was chosen such that the power at the fundamental frequency was identical in all cases. In each presentation, which follows the model of figure 4.3, the probability (p) of the P-unit firing has been plotted against the phase difference (t_1-t_2) of the firing of the two T-units (diagram in center). Whereas the p/t graphs in (b) are closed and thus reveal no sense of rotation, those obtained for clipped S_1 signals in (c) and (d) open up and show opposite senses of rotation (arrows) for opposite signs of Df. In addition, the rotation observed for a given sign of Df also reverses with a reversal of the polarity of the clipping. (From Heiligenberg and Partridge 1981)

Depending on the particular pair of T-units chosen for generating such graphs, the correct polarity of the EOD mimic may either yield the correct or the incorrect sense of rotation. But in every case, it reverses for a given sign of Df as the polarity of the EOD mimic is reversed, and the area formed by the loops of these graphs is always small. It appears to be a matter of chance whether the net contribution from all receptors yields correct or incorrect JARs, and slight fluctuations in the state of receptors appear to be capable of tipping the balance. The identical-geometry condition is never encountered under natural conditions as the sources for the two interfering EODs are always different, and the animal is obviously not equipped for determining the sign of Df if the two EOD sources are identically oriented.

It should be emphasized here that the experimental conditions necessary for discrimination of the sign of Df by higher-order neurons in the torus semicircularis are the same as those required for eliciting the JAR. As we shall discuss later, these neurons fail to discriminate the sign of Df under the identical-geometry condition. When we tested such neurons under this condition, they discriminated the sign of Df, although relatively poorly, when the EOD mimic was clipped as in the experiments of figure 4.8, and they again reversed their response as a function of the sign of Df when the polarity of the clipped EOD mimic was reversed (Heiligenberg and Partridge 1981).

THE ELECTROSENSORY LATERAL LINE LOBE

The response properties of electrosensory neurons can be tested by experimental designs previously described in the context of behavioral studies. Amplitude and phase of a sine wave signal can be modulated separately or jointly in order to learn whether a given neuron responds to one or the other form of modulation or to a particular pattern of joint modulations. The two-compartment chamber shown in figure 3.6 allows us to determine whether the receptive field of a neuron sensitive to amplitude modulations lies on the head or on the trunk. For a neuron sensitive to phase modulations between the signal at the animal's head and the signal at the animal's trunk, excitatory and inhibitory ranges of phase values can be determined by systematically shifting the phase of a sine wave applied to the head with reference to an identical sine wave applied to the trunk. In this manner, phase modulations can be generated in the absence of amplitude modulations. While the two-compartment chamber in figure 3.6 is convenient for the testing of neurons with pure phase modulations, it limits us to comparing the phases of head and trunk. Unfortunately, it is technically too difficult to build a two-compartment chamber for independent stimulation of the two sides of the fish, since current leakage between two lateral chambers cannot be eliminated sufficiently.

In order to determine the approximate location of receptive fields for a cell involved in the comparison of signal phases, one may suspend a fish freely in the center of a larger tank and surround it with a circular array of electrodes for the presentation of jamming stimuli. Modulations in differential phase are strongest between points on the body surface which are antipodal with regard to the current vector of the jamming stimulus, such as the two sides of the body exposed to a transverse jamming field as shown in figure 3.8. By presenting a jamming stimulus field at different orientations with respect to the fish's body axis, one can determine the optimal orientation for a given neuron. Phase modulations can then be eliminated by no longer presenting the jamming stimulus through separate sets of external electrodes and instead adding it electronically to the EOD substitute. This identical-geometry condition causes all points of the body surface to experience the same mixing ratio between the two signals. By switching between the identical-geometry and differential-geometry conditions, one can determine whether a given neuron is sensitive to amplitude modulations alone or whether it is sensitive to phase modulations as well. In the following, further details of such experimental procedures will be given with the presentation of data.

The primary afferents of electroreceptors project to four somatotopically ordered maps of the ELL in the hindbrain (see figure 4.1).

Therefore, these maps preserve the spatial order of electric signals on the body surface. Whereas the primary afferents of the ampullary receptors, which code low-frequency electric signals, innervate only the most medial map, each primary afferent of a tuberous receptor sends collaterals to the three remaining maps, the centromedial, the centrolateral, and the lateral map (see figures 3.1, 4.1; Carr et al. 1982, Heiligenberg and Dye 1982). That information from tuberous receptors should be represented in triplicate has long puzzled anatomists and physiologists, and some possible functional as well as evolutionary interpretations will be offered later in this chapter.

Separate processing of phase and amplitude information

The structural organization of the ELL allows for separate processing of phase and amplitude information provided by T-units and P-units, respectively (figure 4.9). A spherical cell receives input from T-units within its receptive field via electrotonic synapses. Maler et al. (1981) proposed on the basis of ultrastructural studies that the narrowness of the initial segment of the spherical cell's axon should offer an electrical resistance sufficiently high that the arrival of an action potential from a single afferent would be unlikely to trigger an action potential in the spike-initiating zone of the axon. Rather, a nearly synchronous arrival of several afferent action potentials should be required to bring the spike-initiating zone of the spherical cell to threshold. This hypothesis has been examined by intracellular recordings from spherical cells.

After the amplitude of the electrical signal substituted for the silenced EOD of a curarized fish has been lowered sufficiently, T-units are no longer driven in synchrony and begin to fire irregularly. Single action potentials arrive at the spherical cell at all phases of the sinusoidal stimulus, but their postsynaptic potentials fail to initiate action potentials in the spherical cell. As the stimulus amplitude is raised, the postsynaptic potentials in the spherical cell aggregate at a specific phase of the stimulus cycle and fuse into larger potentials which eventually suffice to trigger action potentials (figure 4.10). Thus, spherical cells appear to be insensitive to individual afferent signals that arrive out of synchrony with the rest of the signals from their receptive field. Consequently, a single receptor, firing out of phase with its near neighbors, will hardly introduce additional variability in the timing of action potentials of the spherical cell; it fires only in response to a postsynaptic potential that reflects the averaged arrival time of several afferent signals. Therefore, spherical cells code the phase of the stimulus with less jitter than do individual T-unit afferents. If one measures the standard deviation of the latency of action potentials with reference to the zero-crossing of a stimulus of normal intensity, generally values in the range of 10 to 40 μs are found for T-unit afferents, while values almost three times smaller are obtained at the level of lamina 6, the target of projections of the spherical cells (figure 4.11). For both classes of neurons, an increase in stimulus amplitude reduces the jitter in the timing of their action potentials (Carr et al. 1986a).

P-unit afferents form excitatory synapses on the basal dendrites of basilar pyramidal cells. These afferents also excite granule cells which, in turn, inhibit nonbasilar pyramidal cells (figure 4.9). As a consequence, a rise in P-unit firing, which reflects a rise in stimulus amplitude, will excite basilar pyramidal cells directly and inhibit nonbasilar pyramidal cells indirectly. Conversely, a fall in stimulus amplitude releases nonbasilar pyramidal cells from inhibition and causes an increase in their rate of firing. The excitation of basilar pyramidal cells, which are also referred to as *E-units*, thus signals a rise in the stimulus amplitude within their receptive field, while the excitation of non-basilar pyramidal cells, which are also referred to as *I-units*, signals a fall in stimulus amplitude. These two classes of pyramidal cells can be compared with "on" and "off" cells known in visual systems (Bastian and Heiligenberg 1980a, Saunders and Bastian 1984).

Behavioral consequences of pyramidal-cell dynamics

While the spherical cells of the ELL follow modulations in signal phase instantly, the pyramidal cells code modulations in signal amplitude with considerable delays (figure 4.12). If amplitude is modulated sinusoidally and at a rate between 2 and 8 Hz, an E-unit

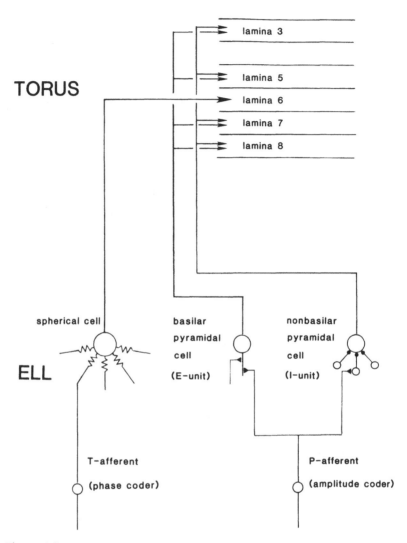

Figure 4.9
The organization of the ELL provides separate substrates for the processing of phase information and amplitude information. Primary afferents from T-type receptors, or *phase coders*, form electrotonic synapses with spherical cells, and a single spherical cell may receive inputs from several T-afferents originating within its receptive field on the body surface. Primary afferents from P-type receptors, or *amplitude coders*, form excitatory synapses on the basilar dendrites of basilar pyramidal cells, or *E-units*, and also excite granule cells which, in turn, inhibit nonbasilar pyramidal cells, or *I-units*. As a consequence of these connections, E-units are excited by a rise in

stimulus amplitude, while I-units fire in response to a fall in stimulus amplitude. Whereas the spherical cells project exclusively to lamina 6 of the torus semicircularis, the pyramidal cells project to various laminae above and below lamina 6. All projections are topographic so that the somatotopic order of electrosensory information is maintained to the level of the torus. Filled triangles indicate excitatory synapses, and filled circles indicate inhibitory synapses. This diagram does not reflect the center-surround organization of the receptive fields of pyramidal cells, which will be addressed in the more detailed representation of figure 4.15.

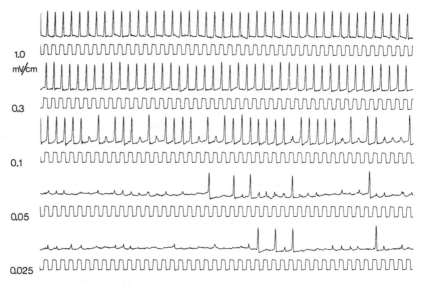

Figure 4.10
An intracellular recording from a spherical cell in the ELL demonstrates that individual postsynaptic potentials (psps, small depolarizations in lower records), generated by the arrival of desynchronized action potentials in T-unit afferents, are insufficient to trigger action potentials. As the stimulus intensity is increased, however, individual psps fuse into larger potentials due to increasing recruitment and synchronization in the arrival of action potentials in T-unit afferents (upper records). With near-natural stimulus amplitudes, these fused psps become sufficiently large to trigger a spike reliably on each stimulus cycle (top two records), and these spikes occur at a fixed phase within the stimulus cycle. The amplitude of the stimulus, measured near and perpendicularly to the head surface, is given at the left of each record, with the value at the top reflecting the amplitude of the natural EOD. A square-wave signal, marking the cycles of the stimulus (170 Hz), is shown underneath each record. The size of the action potentials is approximately 60 mV.

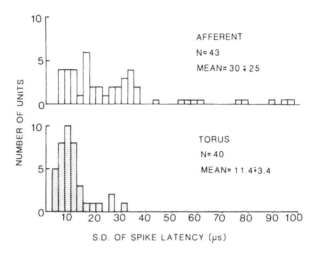

Figure 4.11
The jitter of phase-coding neurons can be measured by the standard deviation of their spike latencies with reference to a fixed point of the stimulus cycle. Standard deviations of T-unit afferents largely fall into the range between 10 and 40 μs (upper histogram), while standard deviations of units in lamina 6 of the torus are approximately three times smaller (lower histogram). Lamina 6 contains the efferent axons of spherical cells, whose somata lie in the ELL and receive input from T-afferents, and the giant cells, which receive input from the spherical cells. These two classes of signals cannot be distinguished by their action potentials recorded in lamina 6, and, therefore, the data have been pooled in the lower histogram. All latency measurements were taken from stable intracellular recordings with action-potential heights of at least 60 mV and a noise level of less than 1 mV. A sinusoidal EOD substitute, S_1, was applied as shown in figure 3.2 and adjusted to yield a nearly normal signal amplitude of 1 mV/cm measured at the surface of the head. The latencies of action potentials were measured at the steepest section of their ascending slope, with a resolution of 0.1 μs, and in reference to the cycle of the function generator supplying the S_1 signal. (After Carr et al. 1986a)

is recruited maximally during the late rise of the amplitude and remains active at the beginning of the subsequent fall of the amplitude. Similarly, an I-unit, recruited during the fall of the amplitude, may still fire while the amplitude begins to rise again. This inertia in the response of pyramidal cells becomes even more obvious at still higher modulation rates so that, at a rate higher than 25 Hz, E-units fire during the fall of the amplitude and I-units fire during the rise (figure 4.12).

This inertia in the response of pyramidal cells has plausible behavioral consequences. First, it could contribute to the phenomenon that the strength of the JAR falls off for magnitudes of Df beyond 8 to 10 Hz. If it is true that a fish recognizes the sense of rotation of a graph in the |S|/H plane by the differential recruitment of E-units and I-units to the right and left of phase zero (figure 4.13), then it should fail to determine the correct rotation for sufficiently high rates of modulation. Namely, due to the increasing lag in the response of E- and I-units, the maximal recruitment of these neurons will eventually occur on the wrong side of the phase axis. For example, for a clockwise rotation, the peak activity of an E-unit may no longer occur for phase advances but more and more for phase delays as a sufficiently large magnitude of Df is chosen, and this, in turn could be interpreted by the nervous system as a counterclockwise rotation. However, the expectation that a fish might shift its pacemaker frequency in the wrong direction, if only sufficiently large magnitudes of Df were presented, was not fulfilled (Partridge et al. 1981).

A second consequence of inertia in the responses of pyramidal cells is the behavioral response to joint modulations of amplitude and phase that physically lack a sense of rotation. In the two-chamber experiments described in figure 3.7, an unmodulated sine wave was presented to one section of the body, whereas the same signal, modulated in amplitude and phase to yield a circle in the amplitude-phase plane was presented to the other section of the body. To obtain such a circle, it is necessary to subject amplitude and phase to sinusoidal modulations that are 90°, or $\pi/2$, out of phase. However, if amplitude and phase are subjected to modulation

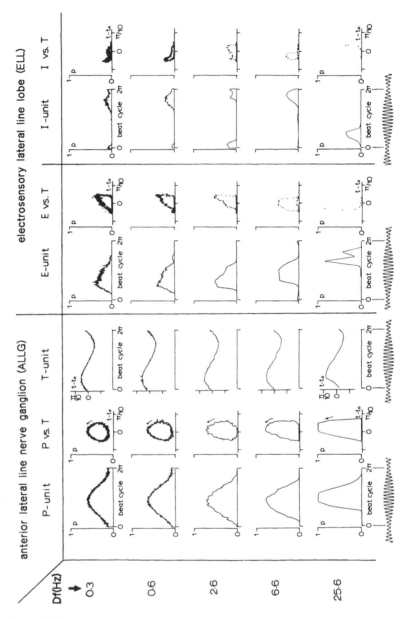

Figure 4.12
Responses of primary electroreceptive afferents, recorded in the anterior lateral line nerve ganglion (ALLG, left), and of E-units and I-units recorded in the electrosensory lateral line lobe (ELL, right), for different positive Dfs, indicated for each line of records on the left. The probability (p) of P-unit firing reflects the modulation of stimulus amplitude during the beat cycle (symbolized at bottom of figure). The relative timing $(t–t_0)$ of T-unit firing reflects the modulation of stimulus phase during the beat cycle. A plot of p versus $t–t_0$ (column "P vs. T" on left) yields a circular graph with coun-

terclockwise rotation for positive Dfs. The firing of spherical cells in the ELL is similar to that of their T-unit afferents and, therefore, is not shown on the right of this figure. For small Dfs, E-units fire predominantly during the rise of the stimulus amplitude, while I-units fire predominantly during the fall of the stimulus amplitude. With larger magnitudes of Df, however, the peak activity of E-units and I-units falls more and more behind. For small positive Dfs, a plot of the probability of E-unit firing versus the relative timing (t–to) of T-unit firing (column "E vs. T" on right) shows predominant E-unit recruitment for positive values of t–to. The opposite distribution of activity is seen in I-units (column "I vs. T" on right). (From Partridge et al. 1981)

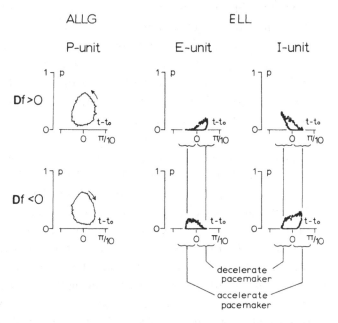

Figure 4.13
The encoding of the sign of Df at the level of primary afferents in the ALLG (left) and at the next higher level, in the ELL (right). The magnitude of Df in these records was 0.6 Hz. The plots on the left are constructed as those in the column "P vs. T" in figure 4.12, the plots on the right follow those in columns "E vs. T" and "I vs. T" in that figure, respectively. It is assumed that E-unit recruitment paired with positive values of t–to, and I-unit recruitment paired with negative values of t–to lower the pacemaker frequency, while opposite pairings of E- and I-activity with the respective signs of t–to raise the pacemaker frequency. This simple rule would explain how the animal lowers and raises its pacemaker frequency for positive and negative Dfs, respectively. (From Partridge et al. 1981)

functions that are in phase or 180° out of phase, diagonally oriented lines are obtained instead of circles. Examples are shown in the upper graphs in figure 4.14b and c. Since these lines do not enclose an area and, therefore, have no sense of rotation, and since they represent symmetrical oscillations (in contrast to the streaks used in figure 3.12), they should not elicit a behavioral response. Surprisingly, the animal lowers its pacemaker frequency if the line has positive slope (figure 4.14b), whereas it raises its frequency if the line has negative slope (figure 4.14c). Therefore, the positively sloping line appears equivalent to a counterclockwise rotation in the amplitude-phase plane, while the negatively sloping line appears equivalent to a clockwise rotation.

The answer to this puzzle may be found in the inertia of the responses of pyramidal cells to amplitude modulations. As shown in figure 4.14b and c, a rising line causes E-units to be more active for phase lags and I-units to be more active for phase leads, a pattern which also emerges for a counterclockwise rotation (see figure 4.13, upper set of records). On the other hand, a falling line causes the opposite asymmetry of E-unit and I-unit recruitment, and this corresponds to a clockwise rotation. The behavioral responses elicited by these line graphs indicate that the nervous system of this fish indeed detects a sense of rotation by the pattern of E-unit and I-unit recruitments in reference to the phase of the signal.

Figure 4.9 simplifies the circuitry of the pyramidal cells in that it ignores the center-surround organization of their receptive fields as well as modulatory inputs originating from descending recurrent inputs. These, as well as other details of the ELL circuitry, are not of immediate importance for understanding the JAR and therefore will be treated separately in the next section. Readers not interested in these details may proceed to the section entitled The Torus Semicircularis.

Figure 4.14
(a) Responses of an E-unit and of an I-unit to a sinusoidal, 4 Hz modulation (top) of the amplitude of an EOD substitute (S_1). For an S_1 frequency of 400 Hz, the amplitude modulation cycle (abscissa) would cover 100 S_1 cycles. The ordinates in the lower plots demonstrating neuronal responses show the probability of firing within the period of an S_1 cycle.

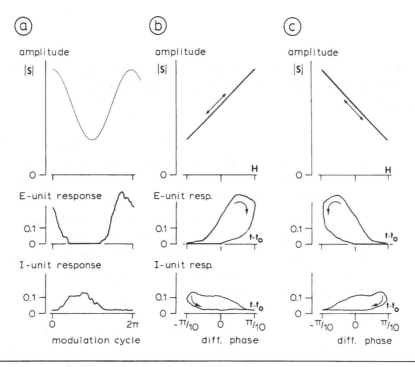

This probability is estimated by the mean number of spikes obtained for this particular S_1 cycle over many repetitions of this amplitude modulation. At a modulation rate of 4 Hz, an E-unit fires maximally during the late rise of the amplitude and continues to fire well into the period of the subsequent fall of the amplitude. A similar inertia is seen in the response of I-units. (b) Responses of the same units during simultaneous modulations of the amplitude of the S_1 (as in a) and of its phase (abscissa). With both variables, amplitude and phase, being modulated by the same sinusoidal function, a plot of amplitude (|S|) versus phase (H) yields a dot travelling back and forth on a straight line inclined 45° upwards (top diagram). If the spike rates of the E-unit and of the I-unit are plotted against the simultaneously recorded phase $(t–t_0)$ of the firing of a T-unit, graphs are obtained that show E-unit activity dominating to the right of phase zero and I-unit activity dominating to the left of phase zero (lower diagrams). This is due to the fact that the E-unit fires predominantly toward the end of the rise in amplitude, while the I-unit fires predominantly toward the end of the decline in amplitude. A similar distribution of E- and I-unit activity would be obtained for a counter-clockwise rotation in the |S|/H plane, i.e., E-unit recruitment predominating on the right and I-unit recruitment predominating on the left (see figure 4.13). As a consequence, the fish lowers its pacemaker frequency in response to the stimulus regimen shown at the top. (c) Same as (b), with the exception that the phase, H, was modulated by the negative of the sine wave that modulated |S|. As a consequence, a straight line is obtained which is inclined 45° downward in the |S|/H plane, and the distributions of E-unit and I-unit activity are reversed with respect to the $(t–t_0)$-axis. A similar distribution of E- and I-unit activity would be evoked by a clockwise rotation in the |S|/H plane, and, accordingly, the fish raises its pacemaker frequency under this condition. Arrows in the lower graphs of (b) and (c) indicate the sequence along which pairs of data points are generated over time. (From Heiligenberg 1986)

DETAILS IN THE CIRCUITRY OF THE ELL AND ITS MODULATION BY
RECURRENT DESCENDING INPUT FROM THE NUCLEUS
PRAEEMINENTIALIS

Structural and functional properties of the ELL have been studied
extensively. Ultrastructural investigations by Maler et al. (1981) had
postulated that the basilar pyramidal cells should be excited by a
rise in stimulus amplitude, while the nonbasilar pyramidal cells
should be excited by a fall in stimulus amplitude. Both predictions
were subsequently confirmed by intracellular labeling of physiologically characterized pyramidal cells (Saunders and Bastian 1984). A
center-surround organization in the receptive fields of pyramidal
cells, again first suggested on morphological grounds (Maler et al.
1981), was confirmed by recording the responses of pyramidal cells
to isolated and combined stimulations at central and peripheral
points of their receptive fields on the body surface (Shumway
1989a). Basilar pyramidal cells, or E-units, are excited by a rise in
stimulus amplitude in the center of their receptive field and are
mildly inhibited by a rise in stimulus amplitude in the periphery
of their receptive field. Opposite responses to the same stimuli are
found in the center and in the periphery of the receptive fields of
nonbasilar pyramidal cells, or I-units. After the original anatomical
studies by Maler et al. (1981) had suggested a strict separation of
the synaptic targets of T-unit and P-unit afferents, ultrastructural
studies by Mathieson et al. (1987) on intracellularly labeled and
physiologically identified afferents modified this description by
demonstrating that T-afferents also send collaterals to granule cells.
The functional significance of this minor overlap of T-unit and P-
unit inputs to the amplitude-coding system is still unknown. Figure
4.15 gives a schematic diagram of all known amplitude-coding cell
types and their connections within the ELL. The descending inputs
to the ELL will be discussed after a brief description of its
projections.

Whereas the spherical cells of the ELL project exclusively to
lamina 6 of the torus semicircularis, the pyramidal cells project not
only to various laminae above and below lamina 6 but also send

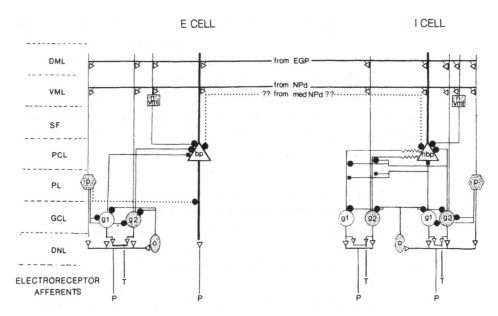

Figure 4.15
A detailed diagram of the amplitude-coding circuitry of the ELL, with a basilar pyramidal cell (bp), or E-unit, on the left and a nonbasilar pyramidal cell (nbp), or I-unit, on the right. Abbreviations for additional cell types: polymorphic cell (p), granule cell of type 1 (g1), granule cell of type 2 (g2), neuron of the ventral molecular layer (n vml), ovoid cell (o). Shaded cells are GABAergic, open triangles represent excitatory synapses, filled symbols represent inhibitory synapses, with filled circles indicating GABAergic inhibition and filled squares indicating non-GABAergic inhibition of as yet unknown nature. Innervation by P- and T-unit electroreceptor afferents is shown at the bottom, and the layers of the ELL are defined as follows: deep neuropile layer (DNL), granule cell layer (GCL), plexiform layer (PL), pyramidal cell layer (PCL), stratum fibrosum (SF), ventral molecular layer (VML), dorsal molecular layer (DML). The dorsal dendrites of several cell types receive excitatory input from the eminentia granularis posterior (EGP) and from the nucleus praeeminentialis pars dorsalis (NPd). GABAergic inhibition of pyramidal cells by the medial NPd and by polymorphic cells is not yet certain (dotted lines). This diagram also demonstrates the center-surround organization of the receptive fields of E- and I-units. An E-unit is excited directly by central input from P-afferents and indirectly inhibited by peripheral inputs via granule cells. An I-unit is inhibited by central inputs and excited by peripheral inputs, with both actions being mediated by granule cells. The role of T-afferent inputs to this amplitude-coding network is still unknown. (From Shumway and Maler 1989).

collaterals to the nucleus praeeminentialis of the midbrain (Sas and
Maler 1983, Carr and Maler 1986). Moreover, the four maps of the
ELL project to four separate maps in this nucleus, and these, in
turn, provide descending recurrent input to the ELL along two separate pathways: one direct pathway, and one indirect pathway via
the eminentia granularis posterior of the lobus caudalis of the cerebellum (figures 4.15, 4.16). These two recurrent inputs have different synaptic targets within the ELL and appear to serve different
functions.

In vitro physiology and immunohistochemical staining of the ELL
have identified the nature of transmitters operating at various sites
in its circuitry (Maler and Mugnaini 1986, Nadi and Maler 1987,
Mathieson and Maler 1988, Shumway and Maler 1989; see figure
4.15). By recording the response properties of neurons before and
after application of agonists or antagonists at selected sites in their
dendritic structure, one can test the suggested functions of specific
connections within the network of the ELL. For example,
GABAergic synapses have been shown to modify temporal and spatial response characteristics of pyramidal cells (Shumway and Maler
1989).

By selective and reversible anesthesia of the indirect recurrent
pathway, Bastian (1986a,b) and Bastian and Bratton (1990) demonstrated that the pyramidal cells of the ELL receive inhibitory input
via this route. This input, which originates in the multipolar cells
of the nucleus praeeminentialis and recruits the granule cells of the
eminentia granularis posterior (see figure 4.15), provides gain control by allowing the pyramidal cells of the ELL to operate over a
wide range of amplitude levels. By causing rapid adaptation to sustained changes in stimulus amplitude, this recurrent input is
responsible for the phasic response properties of the pyramidal cells.
Inhibition appears to be mediated via the polymorphic cells or the
class-2 granule cells. Both types of cells receive excitatory, glutaminergic input from the eminentia granularis of the lobus caudalis at
their dorsal dendrites and form inhibitory, GABAergic synapses on
the pyramidal cells (see figure 4.15). This interpretation has been
supported by Shumway and Maler (1989), who applied the GABA

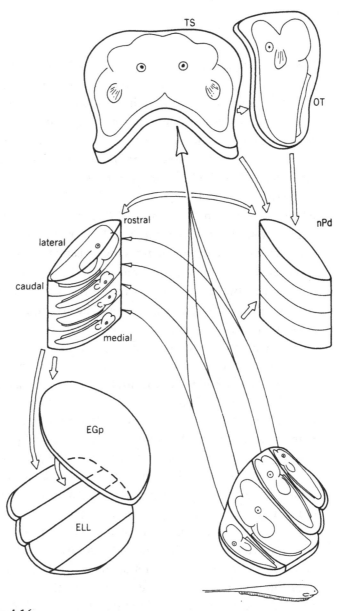

Figure 4.16
Projections and recurrent, descending innervation of the ELL. The four
electrosensory maps of the ELL are preserved separately in their projection
to the nucleus praeeminentialis pars dorsalis (nPd), and the nPd provides
direct and, via the eminentia granularis posterior (EGp) of the lobus caudalis, indirect recurrent input to the ELL. The somatotopic order of electrosensory information is also maintained in a single, but multilayered
body map in the torus semicircularis (TS) which, in turn, projects to the
optic tectum (OT) as well as to the nPd. The projections of the ELL are
predominantly contralateral. (Courtesy of C.E. Carr)

blocker bicuculline to the pyramidal cell layer and obtained changes in pyramidal cell response properties similar to those caused by Bastian's anesthesia of the indirect recurrent pathway.

Whereas the descending input via the indirect recurrent pathway appears to affect the ELL in its entirety by providing overall gain control, the directly descending input, which originates in the stellate cells of the nucleus praeeminentialis, forms focal, topographic projections to the ELL (Maler et al. 1982), and may function as a localized attention mechanism (Bratton and Bastian 1990).

The existence of three separate ELL maps with identical inputs from tuberous electroreceptors has been a mystery, particularly since all three maps display the same basic cytoarchitecture and only show obvious differences in their overall size and in the relative abundance of certain cell types. The arrangement of these maps within the ELL suggests that they originated by duplication of a single ancestral structure, and the lack of obvious qualitative differences in their physiological properties gives the impression that they are still on their way toward further functional specializations. Detailed physiological studies by Shumway (1989a,b), however, have demonstrated quantitative differences between these three maps with regard to the spatial and temporal response characteristics of pyramidal cells. In comparison to the pyramidal cells of the lateral map, those of the centromedial map have smaller receptive fields, have higher incremental thresholds for changes in signal amplitude, and are less sensitive at higher rates of amplitude modulations. The pyramidal cells of the centromedial map thus show better spatial but poorer temporal resolution than those of the lateral map. The pyramidal cells of the centrolateral map, which lies between the lateral and the centromedial maps, show response properties intermediate to those of their neighbors. It is not yet known whether these three maps are of different significance for the control of the JAR. All three maps have just differentiated at the moment when the JAR emerges in juveniles, at an age of approximately one month and at a total body length of approximately 15 mm (Viete 1990).

THE TORUS SEMICIRCULARIS

Earlier extracellular studies of the torus semicircularis had revealed the existence of neurons coding various aspects of stimulus patterns that are critical for the execution of the JAR (Scheich and Bullock 1974, Scheich 1977). In addition to an abundance of neurons sensitive to modulations of stimulus amplitude, other neurons were then found to code modulations of phase differences between signals at separate points on the body surface (Bastian and Heiligenberg 1980a,b). This discovery of a representation of phase information gave strong support to the neuronal theory of the JAR that had been developed strictly on the basis of behavioral experiments (Heiligenberg et al. 1978b, Heiligenberg and Bastian 1980). Eventually, intracellular labeling of physiologically identified cell types then allowed to link the structural and functional properties of neurons and to reveal the neuronal network of the torus. The definition of toral laminae presented in the following description is based on the study by Carr et al. (1981) and differs from that given by Scheich and Ebbesson (1981, 1983).

Differential-phase computation in lamina 6

The phase-coding and amplitude-coding cells of the ELL project to separate targets in the torus semicircularis of the midbrain. Whereas the spherical cells only innervate lamina 6, both types of pyramidal cells project to various laminae above and below lamina 6 (see figure 4.9). Differential-phase information is computed within lamina 6, and differences in the timing of zero-crossings between signals at any two points of the body surface can be encoded by this network (figure 4.17).

By studying the ultrastructure of intracellularly labeled and physiologically characterized neurons of lamina 6, Carr et al. (1986b) were able to demonstrate that the axons of spherical cells invade lamina 6 in somatotopic order and synapse electrotonically on the somata of giant cells and nearby dendrites of small cells. Giant cells receive inputs from several spherical cells representing a given receptive field on the body surface, and they respond to a suffi-

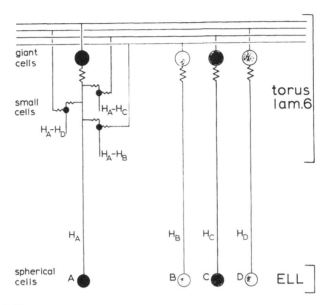

Figure 4.17
Lamina 6 of the torus semicircularis contains a network for the computation of differential phase between any two points on the body surface. The
spherical cells in the ELL (see figure 4.9) receive somatotopically ordered
information about the phase, i.e., the timing of zero-crossings, of electric
signals on the body surface, and they relay this information, H_A, H_B, . . . ,
in a topographic projection to lamina 6 of the torus by synapsing on the
somata of giant cells and the dendrites of nearby small cells. Giant cells,
in turn, relay the phase-locked spikes of spherical cells through their large
axonal arbors to wide areas of lamina 6, and their axonal collaterals synapse
on the somata of small cells, which apparently can accommodate only a
single large synapse of this kind. Therefore, a small cell is controlled by
inputs from two sources: the input at its dendrites is derived from the
point on the body surface represented at its location in lamina 6 (point A
in this example), while the input at its soma originates from the point
represented at the location of the giant cell soma whose axon collateral
forms this contact (point B, for example). Small cells fire intermittently,
and their rate of firing is controlled by the differential timing of their two
inputs. Giant cells receive inputs from several spherical cells within a
receptive field, and only fire in response to a nearly synchronous arrival of
spikes from several spherical cells. For clarity, only a single spherical cell
is shown to contact a giant cell in this diagram. (After Carr et al. 1986b)

ciently synchronous arrival of action potentials on several input lines by firing a single action potential (Carr et al. 1986a). In this regard, the mechanism of spike generation resembles that of the spherical cells in the ELL (see figure 4.10). Giant cells relay their phase information to the representations of many different points of the body surface by sending an extensive axonal arbor across wide areas of lamina 6. Their axon collaterals synapse in apparently random order on the somata of the small cells, and the size of their synapses allows only a single axon to contact any small-cell soma. Therefore, a given small cell receives information about the timing of zero-crossings of signals at two points on the body surface: through its dendrites, it receives input from the point represented at its location within lamina 6 (point A in figure 4.17), whereas on its soma it receives input from the point represented by the location of the soma of the particular giant cell which has established contact via its axon collateral (point B in figure 4.17, for example).

Responses of two small cells to phase modulations between head and trunk are shown in figure 4.18. A more detailed analysis of a third neuron in figure 4.19 shows that it is exclusively sensitive to phase modulations. Finally, figure 4.20 demonstrates that a small cell is spontaneously active in the absence of phase modulations, whereas, in the presence of phase modulations, one range of phase values is excitatory, while the neighboring ranges are inhibitory. Small cells thus sharpen the transition across a critical point on the phase axis by switching from excitation to inhibition. Additional data in figure 4.20 show that a small cell can even discriminate stationary phase values, although its response is crisper when phase is modulated swiftly.

The degree of phase modulation between any two points, A and B, on the body surface depends on the orientation of the jamming field. With A and B lying on opposite flanks, for example, the modulation in the differential phase between their signals will be maximal if the jamming field is oriented perpendicularly to the trunk of the fish (see figure 3.8), whereas the phase modulation will be minimal if the jamming field is oriented longitudinally to the fish. All small cells at the location in lamina 6 representing point

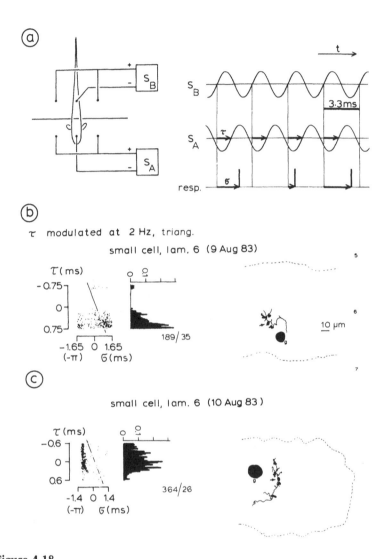

Figure 4.18
Responses of two small cells in lamina 6 to modulations of differential
phase between head and trunk. (a) Representation of stimulus regimen
applied in a two-compartment chamber as introduced in figure 3.6. A
stationary sine wave, S_B, is offered to the trunk, while a phase-modulated
version of this sine wave, S_A, is offered to the head. τ is the differential-
phase value between the two signals (equivalent to the expression H_A-H_B
used in previous figures), and σ is the timing of an action potential with
reference to the nearest zero-crossing of S_B. τ is modulated by a triangular
wave form at a rate of 2 Hz. (b) and (c) show data of two neurons. The

A on the body surface receive dendritic input from point A, whereas their somatic input originates from individually different points on the body surface, without any apparent order. Thus, for a given orientation of the jamming field, some cells at this location will, by virtue of their particular somatic input, experience strong phase modulations, while others will experience little or none. As the orientation of the jamming field changes, the pattern of recruitment of the small cells will change accordingly, and a sufficient individual diversity of somatic inputs will insure that there are always some small cells that experience significant phase modulations, regardless of the particular orientation of the jamming field.

The convergence of phase and amplitude information in deeper laminae

As indicated in figure 4.9, amplitude information reaches various laminae above and below lamina 6, and since all laminae are matched somatotopically, vertical connections between them can provided the basis for a joint and spatially congruent evaluation of differential-phase information and amplitude information. Some cells in laminae 5 and 7 have dendritic fields limited to these laminae, and they respond only to modulations in signal amplitude. However, other cells in these layers have dendrites extending deeply into lamina 6, and these cells also respond to modulations in differential phase. This suggests that the small cells of lamina 6 trans-

---

timing of their action potentials is indicated in the diagram on the far left by dots in a plane having τ and σ as coordinates. The maximal values of τ are ±0.75 ms and ±0.6 ms, respectively. The straight lines indicate the set of points with $\tau = \sigma$. Dots on a profile parallel to this line reflect firing phase-locked to S_A, while dots lined up along a vertical trace, as in (c), reflect firing phase-locked to S_B. The histograms in the center of (b) and (c) show the relative rate of firing as a function of τ, with a bin width of 10 μs and the range of the τ-axis being the same as that in the scattergram on the left. The notation m/n (m and n being integers) gives total number of spikes per total number of phase modulation cycles. Whereas the neuron in (b) is excited by a delay of the signal at the head, the neuron in (c) is excited mainly by an advance. The drawings on the right show a camera lucida tracing of the small cell recorded and the nearest giant cell soma (g). Dashed lines indicate the border of lamina 6. The arrow points to the soma of the small cell. (From Heiligenberg and Rose 1985)

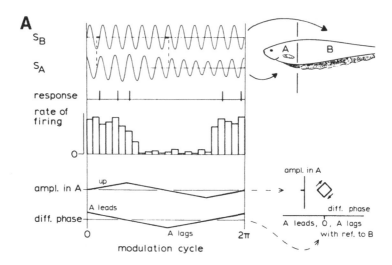

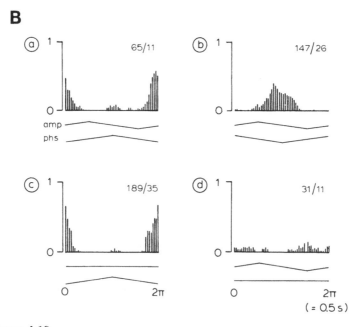

Figure 4.19

Responses of a small cell in lamina 6 to simultaneous modulations of the amplitude and phase of a sine wave (S_A) offered to the head, in reference to the unmodulated sine wave (S_B) offered to the trunk. Part A of this figure shows the experimental procedure and definition of variables. Triangular modulation functions were used instead of sinusoidal functions. For clarity, mit information to dendrites reaching into this layer from below and from above (figure 4.21).

Neurons of lamina 5 and 7 project to deeper laminae of the torus, most prominently to lamina 8c, and some project to targets outside the torus, such as the tectum, the lateral mesencephalic reticular area, and the nucleus praeeminentialis (figure 4.22).

Neurons of lamina 5 and 7 projecting to deeper laminae of the torus apparently relay phase and amplitude information to a variety of higher-order neurons in these laminae. We find neurons responding only to phase modulations (figure 4.23), only to amplitude modulations (figure 4.24), and to both forms of modulations (figure 4.25).

Since the stimulus regimen used in figure 4.25 relies on the normal interference of two sine wave signals, S_1 and S_2, it cannot produce phase modulations independently of amplitude modulations. Independent manipulation of phase and amplitude information is required in order to determine how the neuron responds to either form of modulation alone as well as to particular combinations of both. The two-compartment chamber arrangement pre-

---

a smaller than normal number of carrier cycles has been plotted over the period of the modulation cycle. Clockwise rotations in the amplitude/phase plane (lower right) reflect a negative Df and cause a rise of the pacemaker frequency. The histogram in the center reflects the activity of a hypothetical neuron excited either by a rise in the amplitude of the signal at the head or by a lead of its phase. An independent manipulation of these two variables allows one to discriminate between these alternatives. Part B of this figure provides data of the small cell tested in this regimen. The normalized histograms have a bin width of 10 ms, and the modulation symbols for amplitude and phase shown underneath are explained in A. The modulation rate was 2 Hz. The ordinates show the mean number of spikes per 10 ms bin. A comparison of (a) and (b) shows that this neuron is excited by a phase lag of the signal at the head, regardless of the simultaneous modulation in amplitude. (c) shows that this is true even in the absence of an amplitude modulation. (d) shows that this neuron is not driven by amplitude modulations alone. Whereas the pattern of joint amplitude and phase modulations in (a) reflects a counterclockwise rotation in the amplitude/phase plane, the pattern in (b) reflects a clockwise rotation. The notation n/m gives total number of spikes over total number of modulation cycles. The depths of phase and amplitude modulations correspond to those generated by a jamming signal of one-third of the fish's own signal amplitude. (From Heiligenberg and Rose 1985)

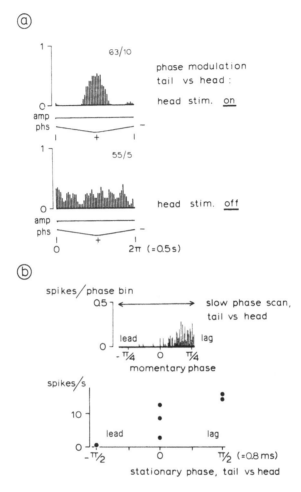

Figure 4.20
Responses of a small cell in lamina 6 to phase modulations of the signal
at the trunk (here referred to as "tail") with reference to that at the head.
(*a*) Presentation as in figure 4.19 *B*, with no amplitude modulation applied.
The phase modulation covers a range from $-\pi/4$ to $+\pi/4$ and has a rate of
2 Hz. This neuron fires in response to a phase lag of the signal applied to
the trunk and is silent otherwise (upper diagram). With the reference signal
at the head silenced, the neuron fires spontaneously throughout the modulation cycle (lower diagram). (*b*) The same cell also responds to phase
modulations 10 times slower than those in *a*) (upper diagram), and it can
even discriminate stationary phase differences (lower diagram). Positive
phase values represent phase lags of the signal at the trunk. Phase values
in the lower diagram were held constant for at least 3 s for each data point.
(From Heiligenberg and Rose 1985)

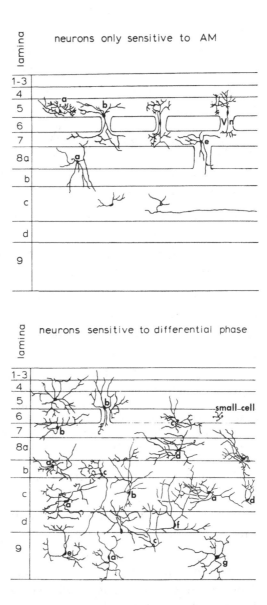

Figure 4.21
Top: Laminar distribution of toral cell types found to be sensitive to amplitude modulations but not to phase modulations under any orientation of the jamming stimulus. Camera lucida drawings of cells filled with Lucifer yellow. The neuropil of lamina 6 is penetrated by vertical neuropil bundles (Vn), which contain afferent and efferent fibers as well as a characteristic cell type. Lower-case letters refer to cell types identified by Carr and Maler (1985) in Golgi material. Bottom: Laminar distribution of cell types sensitive to differential phase. Cells in laminae 5 and 7 send dendrites into lamina 6. One unlabeled type of cell in lamina 5, shown at the left, is not yet known from Golgi studies. (From Rose and Heiligenberg 1985a)

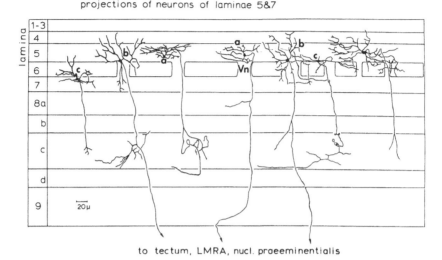

projections of neurons of laminae 5&7

to tectum, LMRA, nucl. praeeminentialis

Figure 4.22
Neurons of laminae 5 and 7 with axonal collaterals in deeper laminae of
the torus. Some of these neurons also project to various targets outside the
torus, such as the optic tectum, the lateral mesencephalic reticular area
(LMRA), and the nucleus praeeminentialis. Neurons with dendrites in lamina 6 (see figure 4.21, bottom) appear to relay differential-phase information
to deeper laminae, particularly to lamina 8c. Presentation and symbols as
in figure 4.21. Neuron type at the far right is not yet known from Golgi
material. (From Rose and Heiligenberg 1985a)

sented in figure 4.19 overcomes this limitation at least for neurons
that respond to differential phase between signals at the head and
at the trunk. The neuron presented in figure 4.26 responds to a rise
of the stimulus amplitude at the trunk (panel *i*) and is, therefore,
classified as an E-type. Panels *a* and *b* show that the same neuron
is also excited by a phase delay of the signal at the head, which is
equivalent to a phase advance of the signal at the trunk, which is
also the source of its amplitude input. In other words, this neuron
has both E-unit characteristics and "phase-advance" characteristics,
and it is, therefore, maximally excited if a rise in the amplitude of
the signal at the trunk coincides with a phase advance of the same
signal in reference to that at the head (panel *g*). Therefore, this

neuron is classified as an *E-advance* type. The responses to amplitude and phase add almost linearly in this neuron.

Laminae 8b and 8c of the torus contain types of neurons that respond to all possible combinations of amplitude and phase modulations, E-types responding to a rise in amplitude, and I-types responding to a fall in amplitude. In conjunction with their preferred phase states, this yields four types of neurons, *E-advance*, *E-delay*, *I-advance*, and *I-delay*. These four types so far cannot be discriminated on the basis of their morphology. All four types project to the tectum, and more heavily labeled neurons also show finer collaterals in the lateral mesencephalic area (LMRA), some of which appear to head for the nucleus electrosensorius in the diencephalon (figure 4.27). Since collaterals projecting to the diencephalon are very fine, they can hardly be traced if cells have been labeled with Lucifer yellow, which we commonly used in our earlier studies. All too often, the fluorescent label of these fine branches bleached too rapidly to allow proper focussation for photography or tracing in a camera lucida drawing. Recently, we have labeled such neurons by intracellular injection of biocytin (Horikawa and Armstrong 1988), and extensive projections to the complex of the nucleus electrosensorius and even to the thalamus have become visible (Metzner and Heiligenberg 1990, 1991).

The discrimination of the sign of Df is still ambiguous

The JAR requires a discrimination of the sign of Df. Could any of the toral neurons described so far code the sign of Df so reliably that records of a single neuron would reveal the sign of Df unambiguously? The neuron portrayed in figure 4.26 fires above its average level in response to a combination of a rise of the stimulus amplitude of the signal at the trunk and a phase advance of the same signal with reference to that at the head. Both stimulus conditions are fulfilled for a clockwise rotation in the amplitude-phase plane which, therefore, recruits this neuron more strongly than a counterclockwise rotation (compare *g* and *h* in figure 4.26). A clockwise rotation, however, implies a negative Df if the jamming stimulus affects the surface of the trunk more heavily than the surface

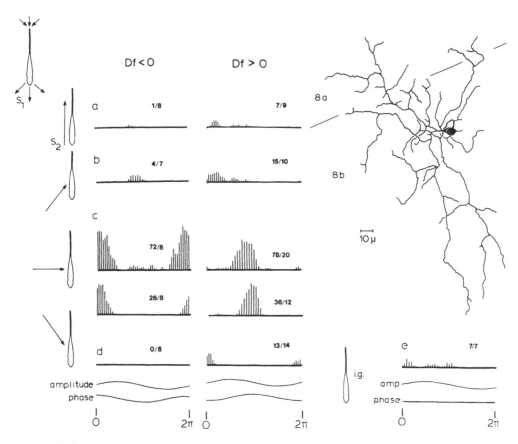

Figure 4.23
Example of a toral neuron excited only by modulations of differential phase. The fish's EOD has been replaced by a sinusoidal signal (S_1) of similar frequency, amplitude and spatial distribution (see inset, upper left: arrows indicate positive current flow). A second sinusoidal signal (S_2) which was either 2 Hz lower (Df < 0) or 2 Hz higher (Df > 0) than S_1, was presented either through the same pair of electrodes used for delivering S_1 (identical geometry condition, labeled i.g. in *e*) or through pairs of electrodes straddling the fish in different orientations (differential geometry condition, in *a* to *d*). The direction of positive current flow of S_2 is indicated by the arrow at the left in each instance. Spike rates are presented in the form of histograms covering the beat cycle. Each bin covers a period of time equal to the duration of three S_1 cycles, which is 10 ms in this case. The height of a bar reflects the probability of a spike occurring in that 10 ms bin. These histograms were smoothed by a gliding weight function, with the weight ratios 1:2:4:2:1. The numbers to the right of each histogram are total number of spikes over total number of beat cycles. Since the beat frequency is 2 Hz, each histogram covers a period of 0.5 s. These histograms are constructed

of the head, whereas it implies a positive Df in the opposite case (see figure 3.5). Therefore, if one wanted to identify the sign of Df on the basis of the degree of excitation of this particular neuron alone, one would also have to know which part of the body surface, head or trunk, is more heavily affected by the jamming signal.

The information provided by toral neurons is further limited in that their excitation depends on the orientation of the jamming stimulus. Local amplitude modulations are maximal if the current lines of the two interfering fields are parallel, and they are minimal if the current lines run perpendicularly to each other. The excitation of a neuron sensitive to amplitude modulations, therefore, depends on the orientation of the current lines of the jamming field within this neuron's receptive field. Since phase-sensitive neurons of the torus compare inputs from two receptive fields on the body surface, they are driven more strongly by the particular orientation of the stimulus that yields maximal modulations in the differential phase between the two receptive fields. A neuron comparing phase inputs from the left and right side of the body, for example, responds more strongly to a transverse orientation of the jamming stimulus, which causes maximal modulation in the differential phase between left

---

with reference to the pattern of the amplitude modulation. Therefore, histograms of opposite signs of Df have opposite phase modulations, and a unit which is sensitive to the timing of the signal in one part of the body relative to the timing of the signal in another part of the body will respond maximally in different sections of the beat cycle for positive and negative Dfs. For this reason, such neurons are also called "sign-sensitive." This multipolar neuron of lamina 8b (see camera lucida drawing of Lucifer-labeled neuron with soma in lamina 8b at right) was driven only weakly by pure amplitude modulations (e, note that no modulations of differential phase occur under the i.g. condition). However, the unit responded vigorously when the S_2 was presented transversely, which suggests that it is driven by differential phase modulations between the two sides of the body (c, two replications of experiment). The amplitude and phase functions at the bottom of the columns of histograms indicate amplitude and phase modulations (phase advance is up) at all points in space where the positive current vectors of S_1 and S_2 form acute angles. For all points where these vectors form obtuse angles, these functions must be shifted by half a beat cycle (see figure 3.8). This neuron fired maximally during a phase advance of the signal received by the right-hand side of the body relative to the signal received by the left-hand side (see figure 3.8 for details of a left-right phase comparison). (From Rose and Heiligenberg 1985a)

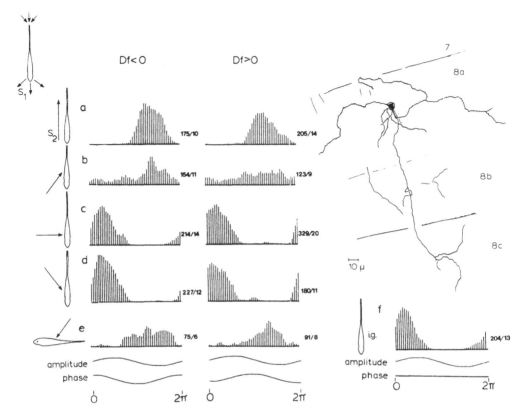

Figure 4.24
Example of a toral neuron excited only by modulations of amplitude (same experiment and presentation of data as in figure 4.23). Each bin represents 10 ms. The soma of the neuron is located in lamina 8a. As can be seen under the identical-geometry condition shown in (f), this neuron responded to a rise in stimulus amplitude (note that all parts of the body surface experience the same amplitude modulation indicated underneath). Under the differential geometry conditions shown in (a) to (e), with the last having an almost vertical orientation of S_2, identical histograms were obtained for positive and negative Dfs at any given orientation of S_2. Therefore, this neuron must have been insensitive to modulations in differential phase. For the following reasons, the receptive field of this neuron was located on the right-hand side of the fish's face. First, in (c) and (d) the S_1 vector and the S_2 vector form acute angles on the right-hand face, and therefore, the amplitude and phase modulations indicated underneath apply to this portion of the body surface. Accordingly, the maximal activity of this neuron coincides with the rise in stimulus amplitude indicated underneath. Second, in (a) the S_1 and S_2 vectors form obtuse angles on the right-hand face and therefore, the amplitude and phase functions indicated underneath must be shifted by half a beat cycle, yielding again a rise in stimulus amplitude while the neuron fires maximally. Third, in (b) the S_2 vector is nearly parallel to the surface of the right-hand face and thus causes a minimal modulation in the amplitude and phase of the signal at this location. (From Rose and Heiligenberg 1985a)

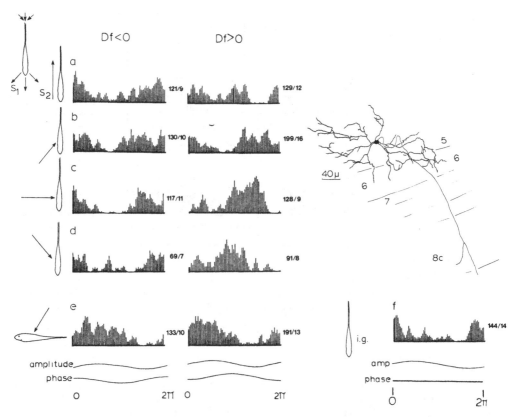

Figure 4.25
Example of a toral neuron responding to amplitude modulations as well as phase modulations (same kind of experiment and presentation of data as in figures 4.23 and 4.24; bin width 8 ms). The soma of the neuron was located in lamina 5. The identical-geometry condition in (f) shows that the neuron is excited by a rise in stimulus amplitude. For the oblique presentation of S_2 in d), the histograms show maximal activity in positions differing by approximately half a beat cycle for positive and negative Dfs. This indicates that the neuron also responds to modulations in the differential phase between the signal on the right-hand cheek and the signal on the left-hand body wall. These points experience maximal modulations in differential phase for the orientation of S_2 in d) (see figure 3.8). Similarly to the neuron shown in figure 4.23, this cell also responds to a phase advance of the right-hand side. (From Rose and Heiligenberg 1985a)

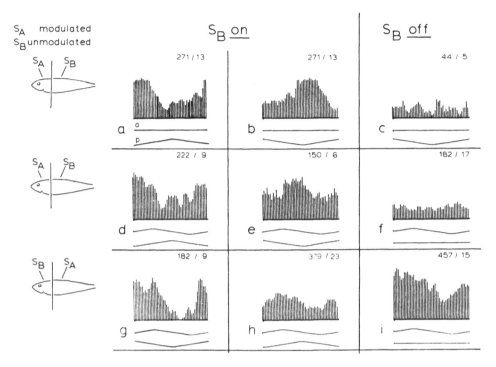

Figure 4.26
The amplitude and phase sensitivity of a neuron can be tested separately in the two-compartment chamber presented in figure 4.19. The modulated sine wave (S_A) is offered either to the head (top two rows) or to the trunk (bottom row), while the unmodulated sine wave (S_B) is offered to the other part of the body (two columns on the left) or turned off (right column). The modulation traces for amplitude (a) and phase (p) underneath each histogram should be interpreted as in figure 4.19. (i) shows that the neuron is excited by a rise of the stimulus amplitude at the trunk, while (f) shows that the neuron does not respond to amplitude modulations at the head. The use of pure phase modulations in (a) and (b) reveals that the neuron is excited by a phase delay of the signal at the head with reference to that at the trunk, and (c) shows that this response requires the presence of the reference signal in the other compartment. Since this neuron does not respond to amplitude modulations at the head (f), panels (d) and (e) show basically the same response patterns as (a) and (b), respectively. A comparison of (g) and (h) reveals that the neuron is entrained most strongly if a rise of the signal at the trunk coincides with a phase advance of this signal with reference to that at the head. (d) starts with a phase *delay* of the signal at the head, which is equivalent to the phase *advance* of the signal at the trunk shown at the start of (g). This neuron was located in lamina 8c. According to the classification of neurons in figure 4.27, this neuron would be considered an "E-advance" type. (From Heiligenberg and Rose 1985)

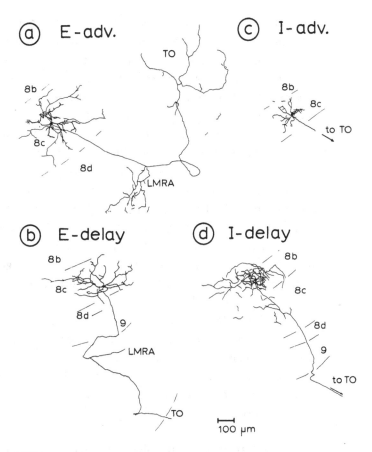

Figure 4.27
Neurons in laminae 8b and 8c of the torus commonly respond to modulations of amplitude and phase. "E-types" are excited by a rise in amplitude,
while "I-types" are excited by a fall. "Advance" neurons are excited by a
phase advance of the same signal, while "delay" neurons are excited by a
delay. Combinations of these response types yield four classes of physiologically distinct neurons of similar morphology. TO is the tectum opticum, LMRA is the lateral mesencephalic reticular area between torus and
tectum. (From Heiligenberg and Rose 1985)

and right (see figure 3.8), whereas it responds poorly to a longitudinal orientation, which minimizes these modulations. As a consequence of this dependence upon stimulus field orientation, the
responses of a neuron may reflect the sign of Df only for particular
orientations of the jamming stimulus and respond indifferently for
orientations perpendicular to the optimum (figure 4.28). Since the
orientation of the interfering stimulus field also determines the
relative contamination of the fish's own signal at different points
of its body surface, it comes as no surprise that, for some neurons,
the preferred sign of Df switches with a particular change in the
orientation of the jamming stimulus (figure 4.29).

The toral cells presented in figures 4.28 and 4.29 discriminate the
sign of Df by a significant difference in their rate of firing. Cells of
this physiological type were first identified through extracellular
recordings by Scheich (1974) and Scheich and Bullock (1974), who
interpreted these cells as "Df decoders." When Rose and Heiligenberg (1985a, 1986a) noted that the sign selectivity of such neurons
depends on the orientation of the jamming stimulus and that, therefore, their responses do not reveal the sign of Df unambiguously,
the label "Df decoder" no longer appeared justified. Rose and Heiligenberg (1985a, 1986a) referred to these cells as "sign-selective"
and argued that large assemblies of such cells could control the JAR
reliably even though individual cells would not provide unambiguous information about the sign of Df (Heiligenberg and Rose 1986).

THE GATING OF AMPLITUDE INFORMATION BY PHASE INFORMATION: A MECHANISM FOR DISCRIMINATING THE SIGN OF Df

Sign-selective cells could discriminate the sign of Df by simultaneous evaluation of amplitude and phase information. As shown in
figure 3.4, a clockwise rotation in the amplitude-phase plane, with
its mean phase at zero, contains a rise in amplitude paired with a
phase advance, while a counterclockwise rotation contains a rise in
amplitude paired with a phase delay. If a neuron were excited by a
rise in amplitude of an EOD-like signal only, or at least more
strongly, under the condition that the same signal also experienced

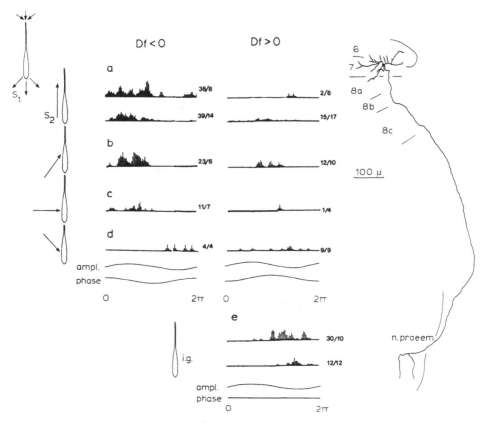

Figure 4.28

A neuron in lamina 7 of the torus shows "sign-selectivity" by firing at a significantly higher rate for one sign of Df than for the opposite sign. This selectivity is limited to the particular orientations of the S_2 field shown in (a) and (b), however. Presentation of data as in figures 4.23 to 4.25, with a bin width of 6 ms. Two sets of data are presented in (a) and (e). The identical-geometry condition in (e) shows that the neuron responds to a drop in stimulus amplitude when phase modulations are absent. This neuron projects to the nucleus praeeminentialis. Fine collaterals projecting to other targets may have been missed due to the rapid fading of the Lucifer label during drawing. (From Rose and Heiligenberg 1985a)

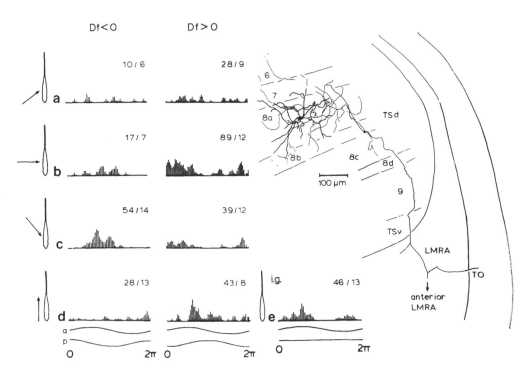

Figure 4.29
The sign selectivity of this neuron in lamina 8a not only depends upon the orientation of the S_2 stimulus, it also reverses with a switch of the S_2 orientation from (b) to (c). Presentation of data is as in figure 4.28. TSd is the dorsal torus, which is electrosensitive. TSv is the ventral torus, which receives mechanosensory and auditory inputs. TO is the tectum opticum, and LMRA is the lateral mesencephalic reticular area. (From Rose and Heiligenberg 1986a)

a phase advance with respect to some reference signal, then this neuron should fire at a higher rate in response to a clockwise rotation than in response to a counterclockwise rotation. This form of gating or facilitation of one input by another input can indeed be demonstrated in the two-compartment chamber paradigm introduced in figure 4.19.

The operation of a neuronal gate

The neuron presented in figure 4.30 was tested by modulating the signal at the fish's head while offering an unmodulated reference

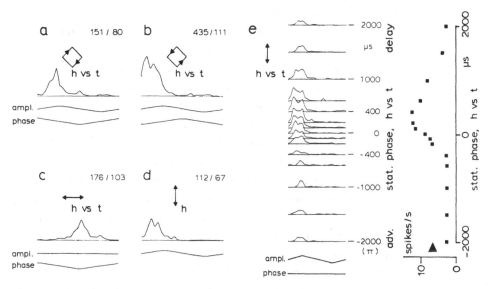

Figure 4.30
The response to amplitude modulations may be gated by the concurrent state of differential phase. Experiments were conducted in the two-compartment chamber introduced in figure 4.19. Normalized spike rates, recorded extracellularly from a sign-selective neuron in the torus, have been plotted as a function of the modulation cycle indicated underneath. A modulated sine wave signal was applied to the head (h), while the unmodulated version of this signal was applied to the trunk (t) or not presented at all. "h vs t" implies that the signal at the head is modulated with reference to that at the trunk. The total number of spikes over the total number of modulation cycles is given for diagrams (a) to (d), and data for several tens of modulation cycles were averaged for each graph in diagram (e) as well. (a) and (b) show data for joint modulations of amplitude and phase resulting in clockwise and counterclockwise rotations. Since the mean phase difference between the modulated signal and the unmodulated reference was zero, these rotations are centered at phase zero. This neuron is excited approximately twice as much by the counterclockwise rotation. (c) A modulation of the differential phase alone revealed a response to phase delay. (d) An amplitude modulation in the absence of the reference signal at the trunk revealed a late response to the rise of the amplitude. (e) Amplitude modulations were applied in the presence of a fixed phase in reference to the unmodulated signal at the trunk. Strongest responses were obtained if the modulated signal at the head had a small phase delay. Since the carrier frequency of the sine wave was 250 Hz, the period of the sine wave was 4 ms long. Maximal phase delays ($+\pi$) and advances ($-\pi$) therefore were +2 ms and −2 ms, respectively. The plot at the far right shows spike rates elicited by amplitude modulations as a function of the stationary differential phase. The triangle indicates the spike rate measured in the absence of the reference signal at the trunk. The depth of amplitude modulations was 30% of the amplitude of the carrier signal. The width of phase modulations was approximately 0.4 ms. All modulation rates were 4 Hz. (From Heiligenberg and Rose 1986)

signal at the trunk, and it was found to respond more strongly to counterclockwise rotations with a mean phase at zero than to clockwise rotations (panels *a* and *b*). The presentation of phase modulations of the signal at the head with reference to that at the trunk showed that this neuron was excited preferentially by a phase delay (panel *c*). Amplitude modulations of the signal at the head in the absence of a reference signal at the trunk revealed that this neuron was excited by a rise in amplitude (panel *d*). When the amplitude of the signal at the head was modulated in the presence of an unmodulated reference signal at the trunk it was found that the response of the neuron strongly depended on the phase difference between the two signals (panel *e*). Highest firing rates were obtained with amplitude modulations combined with small delays of the signal applied to the head. In accordance with this dependence of its response to amplitude modulations on differential phase, this neuron was most strongly excited by a rise in amplitude paired with a phase delay, that is, by a counterclockwise rotation centered near phase zero.

The data in figure 4.30 had to be obtained by extracellular recording since intracellular recordings are not sufficiently stable over the extended period of time necessary for testing this large set of stimulus configurations. Shorter periods of intracellular recordings from sign-selective cells so far have failed to reveal synaptic mechanisms that could account for the gating of one stimulus variable by another. Therefore, figure 4.31 only suggests a mechanism for gating. Alternative mechanisms, based on inhibitory rather than excitatory interactions, cannot be excluded at this point.

The model proposed in figure 4.31 requires two classes of input neurons both of which are abundant within the torus. These are E- and I-type neurons for the coding of amplitude modulations on the one hand, and neurons coding differential phase on the other. The response profile of the phase discriminator depicted in figure 4.31 has been confirmed experimentally by using the two-chamber approach shown in figure 3.6 and by scanning the signal presented to the head with reference to that presented to the trunk (Rose and Heiligenberg 1986b). In this way, a full scan from $-\pi$ to $+\pi$ could

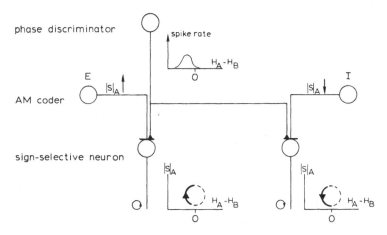

Figure 4.31
A model for the joint computation of amplitude and phase information by
a sign-selective neuron. Information is provided from two areas, A and B,
on the body surface. A phase-discriminator neuron that is excited by small
negative values of the differential phase, $H_A–H_B$ (top), i.e., small phase leads
of area A over B, is assumed to facilitate input from amplitude modulation
(AM) coders for area A to sign-selective neurons. Two classes of AM coders,
E-neurons and I-neurons, are respectively excited by a rise and by a fall in
the local stimulus amplitude ($|S|_A$). As a consequence of facilitation, the
sign-selective neuron on the left prefers a clockwise rotation centered at
phase zero, i.e., a combination of a rise with a phase advance, while the
neuron on the right prefers a counterclockwise rotation. (From Heiligenberg
1987)

be executed. As shown in the example given in figure 4.32*a*, a
neuron sensitive to differential phase fires most strongly within a
limited phase range centered on either side of zero, which is either
an advance (as in the case shown in figure 4.32*a*), or a delay; and
these ranges roughly coincide with those that were shown to be
most effective in the behavioral tests described in figure 3.12. While
the neuron presented in figure 4.32 also responds to modulations
in stimulus amplitude, other phase discriminators respond to phase
modulations exclusively. Furthermore, as one records from such
neurons in the rostral portion of the torus, which represents the
electrosensory surface of the head region, one may find neurons
excited by a phase advance of the signal at the head with reference

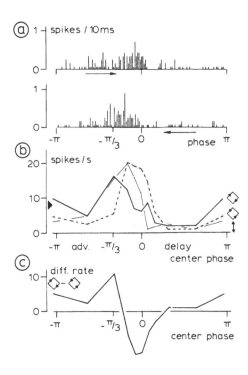

Figure 4.32
The gating of the response to amplitude modulations by differential phase
implies that a neuron may prefer different senses of rotation as a graph is
shifted to different center phases. This neuron was tested in the two-
compartment chamber (figure 4.19), with a modulated sine wave applied
at the head, and its unmodulated version applied as a reference to the
trunk. It was excited by a phase advance as well as by a decline in amplitude
of the signal at the head. (a) A constant modulation of the phase of the
signal at the head with reference to the signal at the trunk. Data for phase
scans at a constant rate, from $-\pi$ to π, are shown in the upper histogram.
Data for phase scans in the opposite direction are shown in the lower
histogram. The total duration of a single scan is 1.25 s. The mean number
of spikes per 10 ms bin, calculated for 12 repetitions, is plotted on the
ordinate. Since a scan is of a constant rate and covers 125 bins of 10 ms,
each bin contains $2\pi/125$ radians, or 2.88 degrees. The period of the EOD
replacement signal was 2.5 ms, and therefore 2.88 degrees correspond to a
shift of 20 μs within the EOD cycle. The mean rate of firing was 13.6
spikes/s. (b) Mean rate of firing in response to stimulus regimens applied
to the head, with given center phase values (abscissa) in reference to the
unmodulated signal at the trunk. Thick line: clockwise rotations, with a
30% amplitude modulation and a peak-to-peak phase modulation spanning

to that at the trunk as frequently as one may find neurons excited by a phase delay instead.

Behavioral consequences of delayed phase information

The mechanism for gating or facilitation suggested in figure 4.31 implies that a neuron preferring a clockwise rotation centered at phase zero should prefer a counterclockwise rotation centered sufficiently far to the left from zero so that the rise in amplitude again coincides with the phase values required for gating. This is demonstrated in the neuron presented in figure 4.32.

Behavioral experiments presented in connection with figure 3.5 suggested that the JAR is driven in a parliamentary manner by a large set of pairwise interactions of receptive fields. A given area, A, was assumed to contribute an accelerating input or a decelerating input as it experienced a clockwise or counterclockwise rotation, respectively, with reference to some other area, B; and the magnitude of this contribution was shown to grow with the depth of the amplitude modulation experienced by area A. A neuronal correlate for this mechanism is offered in the lower half of figure 4.33. It assumes that a sign-selective cell preferring a clockwise rotation centered at phase zero will accelerate the pacemaker in proportion to the depth of the amplitude modulation input, while a sign-selective cell preferring a counterclockwise rotation will decelerate the pacemaker. These sign-selective neurons compute differential phase from two receptive fields, A and B, and receive amplitude information from a third field which is assumed to overlap mainly

---

420 μs. The center of this span is the "center phase" plotted on the abscissa. Broken line: counterclockwise rotations. Thin line: amplitude modulations without phase modulations. Since this neuron was excited by a drop of the stimulus amplitude as well as by a phase advance, it is maximally excited by a counterclockwise rotation centered at phase zero, i.e. where the drop in amplitude coincides with a phase advance. For the same reason, however, it is also maximally excited by a clockwise rotation centered appropriately to the left of phase zero. This observation is summarized in (c), where the differences in spike rates for clockwise and counterclockwise rotations are plotted as a function of the center phase. (From Heiligenberg and Rose 1986)

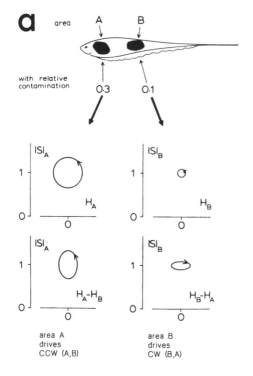

a area

with relative contamination 0.3 0.1

$|SI|_A$ 1 0 H_A 0

$|SI|_B$ 1 0 H_B 0

$|SI|_A$ 1 0 $H_A - H_B$ 0

$|SI|_B$ 1 0 $H_B - H_A$ 0

area A
drives
CCW (A,B)

area B
drives
CW (B,A)

b

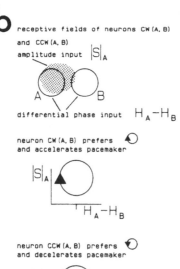

receptive fields of neurons CW(A, B)
and CCW(A, B)
amplitude input $|S|_A$

A B
differential phase input $H_A - H_B$

neuron CW(A, B) prefers
and accelerates pacemaker
$|S|_A$ $H_A - H_B$

neuron CCW(A, B) prefers
and decelerates pacemaker
$|S|_A$ $H_A - H_B$

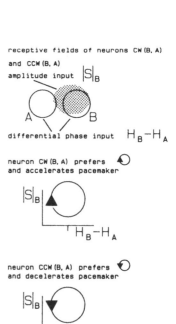

receptive fields of neurons CW(B, A)
and CCW(B, A)
amplitude input $|S|_B$

A B
differential phase input $H_B - H_A$

neuron CW(B, A) prefers
and accelerates pacemaker
$|S|_B$ $H_B - H_A$

neuron CCW(B, A) prefers
and decelerates pacemaker
$|S|_B$ $H_B - H_A$

with one of the two fields. The analysis of sign-selective neurons in the two-compartment chamber paradigm so far does not provide a more detailed description of receptive field sizes and degrees of overlap.

As was pointed out in connection with figure 4.31, a sign-selective neuron appears to recognize a sense of rotation by and-gating a particular form of amplitude modulation, "up" or "down," with a particular state of differential phase, "small advance" or "small delay." As a consequence, a neuron preferring a clockwise rotation centered at phase zero can be fooled into preferring a counterclockwise rotation if its center phase is artificially offset from zero (see figure 4.32). Such offsets do occur naturally because of conduction delays in primary afferent fibers. If a fish is placed in a multicom-

Figure 4.33
The JAR appears to be driven by a parliament of neurons. (a) A fish exposed to a neighbor's EODs with a frequency higher than its own experiences modulations in the local amplitude (|S|) and phase (H) of the electric signal on its body surface that form counterclockwise rotations in the amplitude-phase plane (upper diagrams). However, the fish can only detect differential phases, such as H_A–H_B, and may obtain circular graphs with opposite senses of rotation (lower diagrams, see also figure 3.5 for details). While the counterclockwise rotation in area A is assumed to decelerate the pacemaker, the clockwise rotation in area B is assumed to accelerate the pacemaker. Due to the larger modulation in local amplitude, area A wins in this competition, so that the fish lowers its pacemaker frequency. (b) A set of sign-selective neurons that could control the JAR under the assumption that neurons preferring a counterclockwise rotation (CCW), centered near phase zero, decelerate the pacemaker, while neurons preferring a clockwise rotation (CW) accelerate the pacemaker. Each neuron evaluates the differential phase between two areas, A and B, as well as amplitude modulations within one of these two areas, which is area A for neurons on the left and area B for neurons on the right. The situation depicted in (a) reflects a positive Df, i.e., a neighbor with an EOD of higher frequency so that the fish should lower its own EOD frequency. With the relative contaminations indicated for areas A and B, neurons CCW(A,B) and CW(B,A) will be recruited more strongly than their respective counterparts, CW(A,B) and CCW(B,A). The decelerating effect of CCW(A,B), however, will outweigh the accelerating effect of CW(B,A) due to the stronger amplitude modulation in area A and the ensuing stronger recruitment of CCW(A,B). (From Heiligenberg and Rose 1986)

partment chamber and then restricted to obtain differential-phase information only from two widely separated areas, A and B (figure 4.34), it will shift its pacemaker frequency consistently in the wrong direction. If the input to the more distal area, B, is then given a sufficient phase advance, however, the fish will show a correct JAR (Heiligenberg and Bastian 1980). This phase advance obviously compensates for the larger conduction delays of T-type afferents originating from more caudal regions so that the central representation

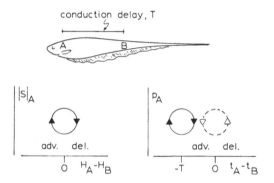

Figure 4.34
Conduction delays in the transmission of phase information may cause incorrect signals for the control of the JAR. With area A being more heavily contaminated by the neighbor's EOD than area B, the graph in the lower left would rotate clockwise for a negative Df and the fish would raise its EOD frequency in an attempt to increase the magnitude of Df. Due to the longer travel time of action potentials originating more caudally, the neuronal representation of the circle is shifted to the left (lower right; p_A is probability of firing of P-type receptors in area A, which codes the stimulus amplitude, $|S|_A$; t_A-t_B is the difference in timing of T-type receptor spikes, which codes the differential phase, H_A-H_B). The fall in stimulus amplitude thus coincides with a small phase advance rather than a delay and thus reflects part of a counterclockwise rotation (dashed circle) which should more strongly recruit neurons with decelerating effects (see figure 4.33). As a consequence, the fish will lower its pacemaker frequency unless additional, stronger and correct contributions from phase comparisons between more closely spaced areas outweigh the wrong contribution originating from the distant interaction between A and B. The contribution from the interaction between A and B can be corrected, however, if the signal in B is given a phase advance sufficient to compensate the delay, T. (From Heiligenberg 1987)

of the circular modulation graph is no longer offset from phase zero (figure 4.34).

Measurements of conduction speeds along afferents from tuberous electroreceptors have shown that afferents from more distant receptor locations have higher conduction speeds than afferents from more proximal receptor locations. This distance-dependent difference in conduction speed, however, is not sufficient for a complete compensation of conduction delays for more distant inputs (Heiligenberg and Dye 1982). Predominance of differential-phase computations between closely spaced receptive fields, which occurs as a direct consequence of the wiring of lamina 6 of the torus (figure 4.17), insures that the fish's JAR is less vulnerable to the wrong contributions from distant-neighbor interactions. No distance-dependent difference in conduction speed is seen in the afferents from ampullary receptors, which only code low-frequency signals without any apparent need for high temporal fidelity (figure 4.35).

PROJECTIONS OF THE TORUS SEMICIRCULARIS: THE SEARCH FOR THE PATHWAY CONTROLLING THE JAR

Intracellular recordings in the torus rarely reveal sign-selective neurons, whereas such cells appear to be more abundant in two higher-order structures that receive information from the torus, the diencephalic nucleus electrosensorius (Bastian and Yuthas 1984) and the tectum opticum (Rose and Heiligenberg 1986a, Heiligenberg and Rose 1987). Little is known about the existence of sign-selective cells in a third major projection target of the torus, the nucleus praeeminentialis of the midbrain.

Since the tectum receives a topographic projection of phase- and amplitude-coding neurons from the torus (Heiligenberg and Rose 1985), it appeared plausible that the tectum could process this information to generate its own set of sign-selective neurons. Such neurons were indeed identified among the projecting cells of the stratum album centrale (figures 4.36, 4.37), and since axonal collaterals of these neurons appeared to head for the nucleus electrosen-

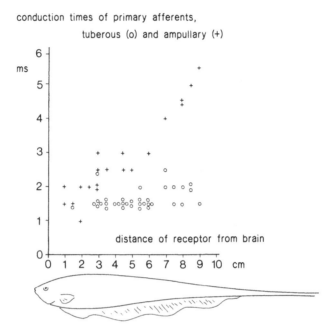

Figure 4.35
Whereas conduction times of primary afferents of ampullary electroreceptors (+) are proportional to the distance between the receptor and the brain,
differences in conduction times of primary afferents of tuberous electroreceptors (o) are partly compensated by higher conduction speeds in afferents of more distant receptors. Spike conduction times were measured by
stimulating individual receptor pores on the body surface of a curarized
fish and recording the latency of the response in the soma of the associated
primary afferent neuron in the anterior lateral line nerve ganglion (as
detailed in Heiligenberg and Dye 1982). The calculated conduction speed
of ampullary afferents is approximately 17 m/s for all locations along the
fish's body. In contrast, afferents of tuberous receptors in the pectoral region
have a conduction speed of approximately 20 m/s, while those of more
caudally located receptors have conduction speeds as high as 50 m/s. All
data in this figure were taken from the same subject.

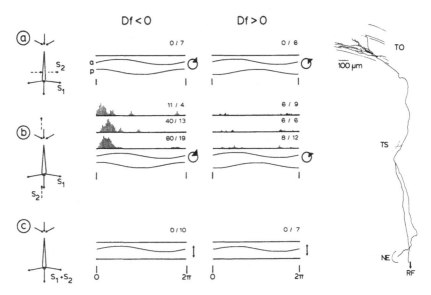

Figure 4.36
Sign-selective neurons are also found in the tectum opticum (TO), although
their presence is not required for the JAR. The neuron in this figure is not
recruited if the S_2 stimulus, which simulates the EOD of a neighbor, is
oriented perpendicularly to the animal (a), whereas it is strongly activated
for a negative Df if S_2 is oriented longitudinally (b, with three replications).
If the EOD substitute, S_1, and S_2 are presented through the same pair of
electrodes (the identical-geometry condition), modulations in differential
phase are absent, and the neuron remains silent (c). The presentation of
data follows the convention of figure 4.29. The camera lucida drawing of
the Lucifer-labeled neuron at the right shows that the main axon projects
to the reticular formation (RF) of the hindbrain, while collaterals project
to deeper laminae of the torus semicircularis (TS) and to the vicinity of the
nucleus electrosensorius (NE). The soma of the neuron is located in the
stratum album centrale (SAC, see figure 4.37). More recent tracing studies
(Keller et al. 1989, 1990) have shown that the tectum does not project
significantly to the NE but rather to more medially located pretectal areas.
(From Rose and Heiligenberg 1986a)

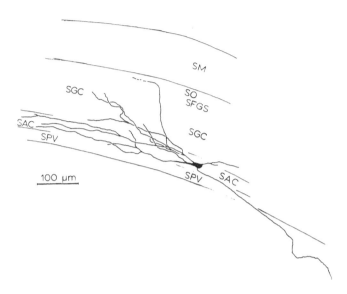

Figure 4.37
Details of the soma and dendrites of the neuron presented in figure 4.36.
The layers of the tectum are: stratum marginale (SM), stratum opticum
(SO), stratum fibrosum et griseum superficiale (SFGS), stratum griseum
centrale (SGC), stratum album centrale (SAC), stratum periventriculare
(SPV). The large projection neurons of the SAC are often multimodal and
commonly respond to the motion of objects (Heiligenberg and Rose 1987).
(From Rose and Heiligenberg 1986a)

sorius, we believed that the tectum was a necessary link in the
control of the JAR (Heiligenberg and Rose 1987). This assumption
was further supported when bilateral lesions of the tectum irrever-
sibly abolished the JAR.

Yet, recent studies by Keller et al. (1990) have shown that those
earlier lesions of the tectum had damaged the efferent fiber tract
from the torus to the nucleus electrosensorius and that more selective lesions of the tectum do not impair the performance of the JAR
at all. Moreover, detailed tracings of tectal projections revealed no
significant projection to the nucleus electrosensorius itself but
rather to pretectal areas in the region medial to that nucleus. Therefore, the sign-selectivity of tectal neurons seems to have no significance for the control of the JAR, and instead appears as a byproduct

of a sensitivity to specific, joint modulations in the amplitude and differential phase of electric signals. As was shown earlier in connection with figure 2.3, moving objects may generate joint modulations in the amplitude and in the phase of the fish's EOD that form curved contours in the amplitude-phase plane, and since the direction of motion along such contours reflects the direction of the motion of the object in space, a sign-selective neuron should also be able to discriminate the direction of object motion (Rose et al. 1987, Rose and Heiligenberg 1986a). The tectum appears to play a major role in the electrolocation of objects. It shows an abundance of neurons sensitive to electrical cues provided by moving objects, and many of these neurons, in addition, also respond to visual and mechanical cues, thus generating a multimodal representation of the environment (Bastian 1982, 1986a; Heiligenberg and Rose 1987).

Whereas sufficiently restricted lesions of the tectum opticum have ruled out its participation in the control of the JAR, small lesions within the complex of the diencephalic nucleus electrosensorius have identified structures that are necessary for the JAR (Keller and Heiligenberg 1989).

THE DIENCEPHALIC NUCLEUS ELECTROSENSORIUS, A SENSORY-MOTOR INTERFACE

Various laminae of the torus semicircularis project to the nucleus electrosensorius (nE) of the diencephalon (Carr et al. 1981), and the loss of somatotopic order associated with this projection suggests extensive spatial convergence (Keller et al. 1989, 1990). Extracellular recordings by Bastian and Yuthas (1984) demonstrated sign-selective neuronal responses within this nucleus. Subsequently, extensive intracellular and extracellular recordings and stimulations by Keller (1988), Keller and Heiligenberg (1989), and Keller et al. (1990) explored the morphology and projections of sign-selective neurons within the nucleus electrosensorius. The data demonstrated significant differences in the response properties of sign-selective neurons in the torus and in the nE.

First, responses of sign-selective neurons of the nE are less dependent on the orientation of the jamming stimulus and, in general,
show a higher degree of sign-selectivity. Most importantly, their
"sign-preference" never changes with the orientation of the stimulus (Keller 1988) (figure 4.38).

Second, sign-selective neurons of the nE are more sensitive to
weak interfering signals, with some of these neurons approaching
behavioral thresholds (Rose and Heiligenberg 1985b). Note that
with a weakening of a jamming stimulus, the depth of amplitude
modulations as well as the width of phase modulations approach
zero. And whereas the most sensitive toral neurons can discriminate phase modulations not smaller than approximately 10 µs (Rose
and Heiligenberg 1986b), neurons in the nE can discriminate phase
modulations as small as 1 µs (Keller 1988).

Third, whereas the firing rate of toral neurons is conspicuously
modulated by the temporal modulations of phase and amplitude
that characterize a beat pattern, the firing rate of neurons in the nE
is less strongly affected by these modulations (see figure 4.43) (Rose
et al. 1988).

Fourth, toral neurons show a large variation in their best beat
rate—that particular beat rate which excites a given neuron most
strongly—although neurons that are tuned to the behaviorally most
effective range of beat rates (2 to 6 Hz) are most abundant (Partridge
et al. 1981). Neurons of the nE show greater preponderance of tuning
to this particular range of beat rates (Bastian and Yuthas 1984).

All of these properties are likely consequences of the extensive
spatial convergence of toral inputs into the nE:

First, a pooling of inputs from toral neurons with individually
different, best jamming stimulus orientations should yield a higher-
order neuron in the nE that is less dependent on this parameter.

Second, since toral neurons reveal a higher sensitivity to small
jamming signals if their responses are averaged over longer periods
of time (Rose and Heiligenberg 1986b), simultaneous averaging over
many such neurons will yield a higher sensitivity immediately.

Third, since individual toral neurons show peak firing rates in
different parts of the beat cycle, the pooled activity of many such

neurons will yield a firing rate distributed more evenly over the beat cycle.

Fourth, with the majority of toral neurons being tuned to beat rates between 2 and 6 Hz, most neurons in the nE should reflect a similar preference for this range.

The response properties of the sign-selective neurons in the nE are thus more similar to those of the JAR itself, lending credence to the notion that this nucleus is a necessary link in the control of the JAR.

By stimulating small clusters of neurons in the nE by iontophoretic application of L-glutamate, Keller and Heiligenberg (1989) were able to identify functionally distinct areas within it. Whereas stimulation of a small dorsal area, nE↑, caused a smooth rise in EOD frequency, stimulation of a more ventrally and rostrally located area, nE↓, caused a smooth fall in EOD frequency. These modulations in frequency showed time courses similar to those seen in the JAR, and selective, bilateral lesions of these areas eliminated the respective frequency shifts from the JAR. These two areas of the nE are thus necessary for the control of the JAR. On the basis of their opposite effects on the pacemaker frequency, one should expect that they receive different inputs from the torus. Whereas the nE↓ should receive inputs predominantly from neurons excited by positive Dfs, the nE↑ should receive inputs mainly from neurons excited by negative Dfs. Intracellular studies are still under way to test this assumption (Metzner and Heiligenberg 1990).

The anatomical organization and cytoarchitecture of the nE have recently been described by Keller et al. (1990), but the understanding of their functional implications requires further intracellular labeling of physiologically identified neurons. In addition to the nE↑ and nE↓, Keller and collaborators have identified a subnucleus, nEb, located rostrally to the nE↓ which contains somata of cells strongly driven by beat patterns, that is, the interference of the animal's own EOD with jamming signals. Many of these cells are highly sign-selective and would appear as plausible candidates for the control of the JAR. Since bilateral lesions of the nEb do not significantly impair the performance of the JAR, however, the role of this sub-

A) ORIENTATION INDEPENDENCE

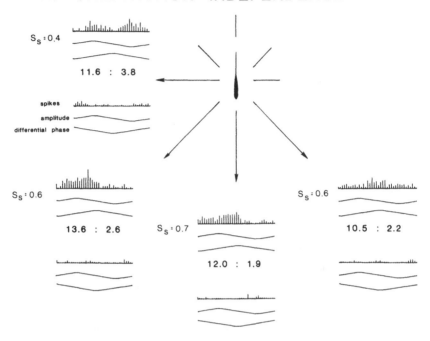

$S_S = 0.4$

11.6 : 3.8

spikes
amplitude
differential phase

$S_S = 0.6$

13.6 : 2.6

$S_S = 0.7$

12.0 : 1.9

$S_S = 0.6$

10.5 : 2.2

B) ORIENTATION DEPENDENCE

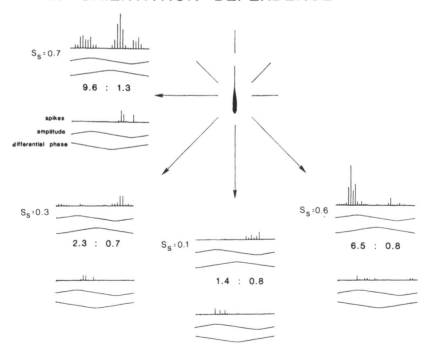

$S_S = 0.7$

9.6 : 1.3

spikes
amplitude
differential phase

$S_S = 0.3$

2.3 : 0.7

$S_S = 0.1$

1.4 : 0.8

$S_S = 0.6$

6.5 : 0.8

nucleus for the JAR is doubtful. An additional area, consisting rostrally of the lateral pretectum and caudally of the nEar, is located medially to the nEb, and it contains cells that respond to interruptions of EOD signals as they occur in the context of courtship and aggression. As original suggested by Hopkins (1974b), such interruptions contain low-frequency components that could be detected by ampullary electroreceptors. We have confirmed this assumption by recent recordings from ampullary electroreceptors and have also found that cells in the nE that respond to interruptions commonly receive inputs from the ampullary system as well (Metzner and Heiligenberg 1991; Heiligenberg et al. 1991). The potential significance of these cells in the context of reproductive behavior will be discussed in chapter 5.

Thus far, only a few cells in the nE↑ and nE↓ have been identified and labeled intracellularly, so that no general statements can be made with regard to the functional properties and projections of cells within these subnuclei. Yet, small injections of tracers indicate that these two areas, as well as the nEb, project to the vicinity of the diencephalic prepacemaker nucleus, which modulates the discharge frequency of the pacemaker in the medulla (figure 4.39). Additional projections to hypothalamic areas probably mediate influences on motivational states by electric social communication (see chapter 5).

Figure 4.38
Sign-selective neurons of the nE prefer the same sign of Df for all orientations of the jamming stimulus, S_2, whereas sign-selective neurons of the torus may change their sign-preference with a change of the orientation of S_2 (see figure 4.29). The neuron in (A) shows a similar degree of sign-selectivity for all orientations, while the neuron in (B) shows some variation. The inset in the upper center of (A) and (B) shows the orientation of the S_2 stimulus field with reference to the fish's body axis. Histograms of the spike rate as a function of the beat cycle have been constructed as in figure 4.29 for each orientation of S_2, with the histogram for the positive Df presented above the histogram for the negative Df and the spike ratios computed for the two signs of Df shown in between. Sign-selectivity (S_s) is defined as log(spike rate for preferred sign of Df $+1$) $-$ log(spike rate for opposite sign of Df $+1$). (From Keller 1988)

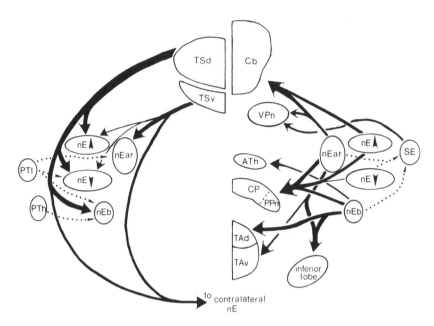

Figure 4.39
Input and output pathways of the nucleus electrosensorius (nE) complex.
As shown to the left, the nE receives input from the dorsal and ventral
torus semicircularis (TSd and TSv), and the dendrites (dotted lines) of some
nE neurons reach as far as to the prethalamic nucleus (PTh) and lateral
pretectal nucleus (PTl). The subnuclei of the nE are the nEb (containing
beat-driven cells), nE↓ (causing pacemaker frequency falls), nE↑ (causing
pacemaker frequency rises), and nEar (acousticolateral region). As shown
on the right, subnuclei of the nE project to the inferior lobe, the dorsal and
ventral tuberculum anterior (TAd and TAv), the prepacemaker nucleus
(PPn), the central posterior thalamic nucleus (CP), the anterior thalamic
nucleus (ATh), the nucleus of the valvular peduncle (VPn), and the cerebellum (Cb). Dendrites of the nucleus subelectrosensorius (SE) reach into
the nE↓. The thickness of connections drawn in this diagram reflects their
relative strength as judged by the number and density of processes. (Courtesy of C.H. Keller)

THE DIENCEPHALIC PREPACEMAKER NUCLEUS

The only neurons that can be labeled retrogradely by injection of HRP into the medullary pacemaker are located in the diencephalic prepacemaker nucleus (PPn; Heiligenberg et al. 1981, Kawasaki et al. 1988a). The PPn thus appears to be the sole source of pacemaker innervation.* Local iontophoretic as well as electrical stimulations of the PPn have revealed two functionally distinct subnuclei: the PPn-G, which elicits gradual frequency rises of the pacemaker frequency, and the more laterally and ventrally located PPn-C, which elicits abrupt frequency modulations (figure 4.40). Whereas the gradual frequency rises are similar to those shown in the JAR, the abrupt frequency rises, or "chirps," which may lead to brief interruptions of the EOD, are signals normally produced in aggression and courtship (Hopkins 1974a,b; Hagedorn and Heiligenberg 1985). HRP transported retrogradely from the pacemaker labels small ovoid cells in the PPn-G and large multipolar cells in the PPn-C.

Intracellular stimulation and labeling of the large multipolar neurons in the PPn-C have shown that single action potentials of these cells are sufficient to elicit a weak form of chirp in the pacemaker (Kawasaki and Heiligenberg 1988). The much smaller neurons in the PPn-G have not yet been recorded intracellularly, but extracellular recordings in their region have revealed small action potentials whose rate is controlled by the frequency difference, Df, between a jamming signal and the animal's own EOD (Rose et al. 1988). These neurons are excited by negative Dfs, which cause a rise in the pacemaker frequency, and are inhibited by positive Dfs, which cause a fall in the pacemaker frequency. This is in accordance with the observation that stimulation of these neurons with L-glutamate also causes smooth rises in the pacemaker frequency.

---

*By using the more sensitive tracer, choleratoxin, we have recently discovered an additional prepacemaker nucleus in the sublemniscal area of the midbrain. Whereas this nucleus induces a sustained depolarization of the relay cells of the pacemaker nucleus in the genera *Hypopomus* and *Sternopygus*, its role in *Eigenmannia* could not yet be determined.

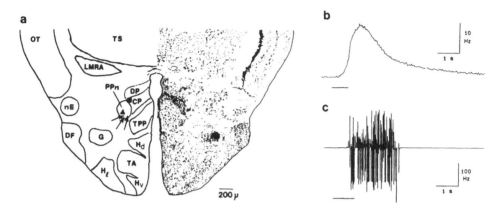

Figure 4.40
(a) Transverse section of the brain of *Eigenmannia* at the boundary between diencephalon and midbrain. The right half was drawn from a 40 μm section stained with neutral red. Neurons of the prepacemaker nucleus (PPn) can be labeled retrogradely by injection of HRP into the medullary pacemaker. Iontophoresis of L-glutamate at two different sites within the PPn elicits different types of EOD modulations: gradual rises (■) and abrupt frequency modulations, or chirps (▲). The region marked by ■ corresponds to the subnucleus PPn-G, while the region marked by ▲ corresponds to the subnucleus PPn-C. Three recording sites for sign-selective neurons are indicated by arrows. These sites were labeled by iontophoresis of alcian blue through a second barrel of the recording electrode. Recordings were probably made from axons that pass through this region of the PPn. (b) Record of instantaneous EOD frequency of a gradual rise elicited by stimulation of site (■) by glutamate iontophoresis. (c) Same for abrupt EOD frequency modulations elicited from stimulation site (▲). The period of iontophoresis is indicated by a horizontal bar in each case. Stimulation and recording sites were marked either by iontophoresis of alcian blue or by small electrolytic lesions in different fish. They were transferred to this representative section by using the surrounding cytology as landmarks. Indicated are the central posterior thalamic nucleus (CP), the diffuse nucleus of the inferior lobe (DF), the dorsal posterior thalamic nucleus (DP), the hypothalamus dorsalis (H_d), the hypothalamus ventralis (H_v), the hypothalamus lateralis (H_l), the lateral mesencephalic reticular area (LMRA), the optic tectum (OT), the glomerular nucleus (G), the nucleus tuberis anterior (TA), the periventricular nucleus of the posterior tuberculum (TPP), the torus semicircularis (TS), and the complex of the nucleus electrosensorius (nE). (From Rose et al. 1988)

In comparison to the sign-selective neurons of the nE, the response properties of sign-selective neurons of the PPn reflect behavioral properties of the JAR to a still higher degree. In three respects, this greater behavioral fidelity appears to result from further neuronal convergence in projections from the nE to the PPn.

First, the recruitment and sign-selectivity of neurons in the PPn is largely independent of the orientation of the jamming stimulus (figure 4.41).

Second, sign-selective neurons that achieve behavioral thresholds in detecting small jamming signals appear to be even more abundant in the PPn than in the nE. The neuron presented in figure 4.42a can still discriminate the sign of Df when the relative amplitude of the jamming signal is as small as 0.001, which corresponds to maximal temporal disparities of less than 1 μs in the associated phase modulations. Behavioral thresholds can be as low as 0.3 μs (Rose and Heiligenberg 1985b).

Third, the firing of sign-selective neurons in the PPn is far less synchronized with the beat cycle generated by the jamming signal than is the firing of neurons in the nE (figure 4.43). The neurons of the PPn fire at a rather steady rate, above their resting level for negative Dfs and below their resting level for positive Dfs. Small beat-related modulations in firing rate are only observed at beat rates lower than 1 Hz, and accordingly, similar weak modulations are seen in the pacemaker frequency at this rate.

A fourth property may not so much reflect neuronal convergence as a more selective projection of nE neurons to the PPn. Although the majority of sign-selective neurons in the nE is tuned to beat rates in the behaviorally most effective range from 2 to 6 Hz, neurons tuned to higher beat rates are found rather commonly in the nE. No such exceptions have been found in the PPn, however, and the preferred beat rate seen at the neuronal level clearly reflects the behaviorally most effective beat rate of the same individual (see figure 4.45; Rose et al. 1988). Presumably, nE neurons tuned to higher beat rates project to neuronal structures involved in the production of chirping; behavioral experiments in the related genus *Apteronotus* have shown that beat rates in the range between 9 and

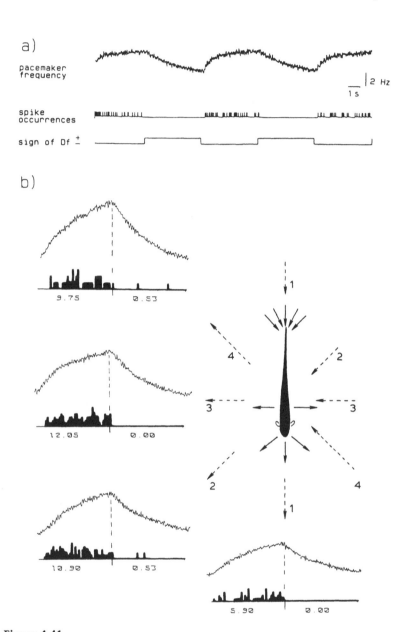

Figure 4.41

(a) Responses of a sign-selective PPn neuron (middle trace) to a jamming stimulus that was alternately 4 Hz lower (negative Df) or 4 Hz higher (positive Df) than the mimic of the fish's own signal. The simultaneously recorded pacemaker frequency showing the JAR is provided in the top trace. All PPn neurons recorded so far were excited by negative Dfs and inhibited

17 Hz are most effective in eliciting chirps, whereas beat rates in the range between 1 and 8 Hz elicit strongest JARs (Dye 1987). This issue will be considered further in chapter 5.

As mentioned in the preceding section, the nE contains two separate areas, nE↑ and nE↓, which control gradual rises and falls in pacemaker frequency, respectively. Behavioral responses to local application to these areas of GABA and the GABA-antagonist, bicuculline, indicate reciprocal inhibition between them. Moreover, sufficiently long stimulation of one of the two areas with L-glutamate eventually leads to a prolonged contraction and suppression of the other (Keller and Heiligenberg 1989). A further mechanism of mutual inhibition could account for the higher sign-selectivity observed at the level of the PPn. In comparison to sign-selective neurons of the torus, those of the nE fire more selectively for either positive or negative Dfs with magnitudes of their preferred frequency difference in the range of 2 to 6 Hz. Yet, quite commonly a neuron tuned, for example, to a positive Df between 2 and 6 Hz may also show a small peak of activity for Dfs between -2 and -6, and this peak may surpass the level of firing for positive Dfs outside the preferred range of 2 to 6 Hz. Therefore, the rate of firing of such a neuron does not reflect the sign of Df unambiguously unless the magnitude of Df is known independently (figure 4.44). Side peaks of this kind are never seen in the response profiles of sign-selective neurons of the PPn (figure 4.45) so that their rate of firing reflects the sign of Df regardless of its magnitude. If neurons tuned to positive Dfs inhibited next-order neurons tuned to negative Dfs and if, analogously, neurons tuned to negative Dfs inhibited next-order

by positive Dfs. (b) A typical sign-selective PPn neuron, excited equally by negative Dfs for all four orientations of the jamming stimulus (broken arrows; solid arrows indicate current lines of the mimic of the fish's own signal). Each spike rate histogram covers the period of the negative-Df presentation on the left and the period of the following positive-Df presentation on the right. The simultaneously recorded EOD frequency is shown above. Numbers underneath the two halves of the histograms are mean spike rates (1/s) for negative and positive Df presentations, respectively. (From Rose et al. 1988)

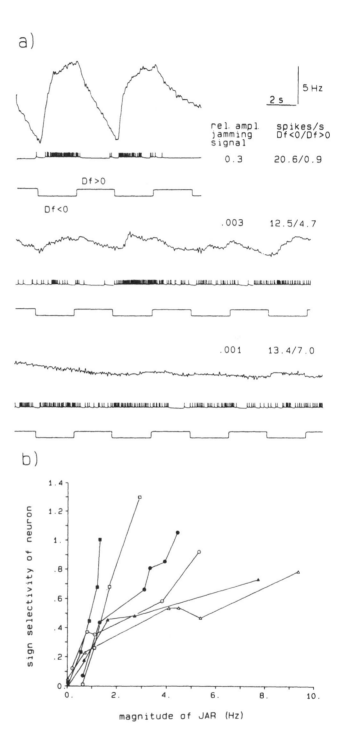

a)

5 Hz

2 s

rel. ampl.   spikes/s
jamming   Df<0/Df>0
signal

0.3   20.6/0.9

Df>0

Df<0

.003   12.5/4.7

.001   13.4/7.0

b)

neurons tuned to positive Dfs, the side peaks depicted in figure 4.44 would be eliminated at the next-order level.

Whereas the nE contains sign-selective neurons excited by positive Dfs as well as neurons excited by negative Dfs, all sign-selective neurons of the PPn recorded so far are excited by negative Dfs and inhibited by positive Dfs. As can be seen in figure 4.42, both excitation and inhibition increase with the relative amplitude of the jamming signal. The nature of this inhibition is still unknown and apparently is not dependent on the action of GABA or glycine (Keller and Heiligenberg 1989). This inhibition can apparently override the excitation by negative Dfs at the single-neuron level. If a fish is exposed to two jamming stimuli, one oriented longitudinally to its body and the other oriented transversely, their effects will roughly add as long as the signs of their Dfs are identical. With the signs of the two Dfs being opposite, however, the inhibitory effect of the particular stimulus with the positive Df will suppress the excitatory effect of the stimulus with the negative Df (figures 4.46, 4.47). This form of nonlinear interaction could be explained if neurons of the nE that are excited by positive Dfs provided a shunting inhibition at the base of the dendrites of sign-selective neurons in

---

Figure 4.42
The effect of attenuation of the jamming signal on the response of PPn neurons and the JAR. (a) A jamming stimulus with a relative amplitude of 0.3, 0.003, and 0.001 of the EOD replacement signal was tested for a single PPn neuron (top, center, bottom panel, respectively). In each panel, top, center, and bottom trace show frequency of EOD, neuronal response, and sign of Df, respectively. Spike rates for negative/positive Df are given at the right of each panel. Although neuronal and behavioral responses became weaker as the amplitude of the jamming signal was attenuated, a marginal sign-selectivity and JAR were still observed at a relative jamming amplitude of 0.001. (b) Relation between magnitude of JAR (defined in figure 3.2) and sign-selectivity (defined in figure 4.38) of neuronal responses with progressive attenuations of the jamming stimulus. Different symbols indicate results from six different neurons. Threshold amplitude for a sign-selective response was determined with a criterion of sign-selectivity of 0.2. Threshold amplitude was less than 0.001 for the neuron in (a), 0.003 for the neurons marked with circles and triangles, and 0.01 for the neurons marked with rectangles. (From Rose et al. 1988)

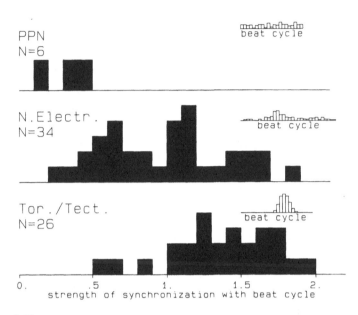

Figure 4.43
The strength of synchronization between spike rate and beat cycle is weakest for sign-selective neurons in the PPn and strongest for such neurons in the torus semicircularis and tectum opticum. An intermediate level is seen in sign-selective neurons in the nucleus electrosensorius. Spike rate histograms (see representative cases in insets at far right) of individual neurons were normalized to yield a mean height of one and were then Fourier analyzed. The amplitudes calculated for the fundamental (beat rate) and first higher harmonic were then added to obtain a measure of synchronization with the beat cycle. The length of the beat cycle was between 150 and 300 ms in each instance, and the Fourier values were normalized to be independent of actual beat cycle length. The number of neurons in each category of synchronization is given by the height of the respective filled bar. The total number, N, of neurons analyzed is given above each histogram. Despite the small number of PPn neurons available for this analysis, the bar histograms differ significantly ($P < 0.0005$, Mann Whitney U-test). The measures of synchronization obtained for the representative spike rate histograms in the three insets are, from top to bottom, 0.13, 0.79, and 1.65. (From Rose et al. 1988)

FREQUENCY DIFFERENCE TUNING

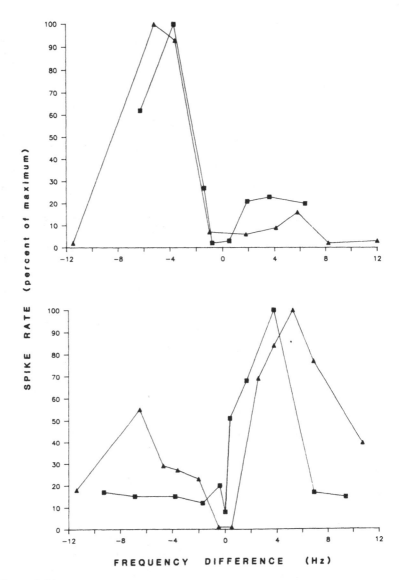

Figure 4.44
Tuning of sign-selective cells of the nucleus electrosensorius to Dfs
between the jamming signal and the fish's own signal. The tuning curves
of four neurons, with their highest spike rate normalized to 100, are shown.
The neurons in the top and bottom diagrams prefer negative and positive
Dfs, respectively. Note that the spike rate of these neurons also show small
peaks for Dfs with a sign opposite and a magnitude similar to that of the
preferred Df. (From Keller 1988)

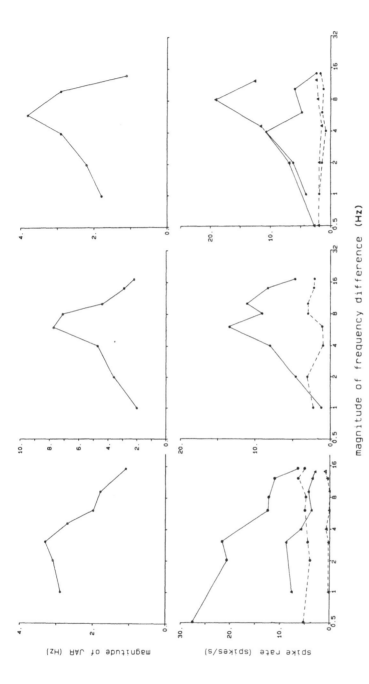

Figure 4.45
Magnitude of the JAR (top panels) and spike rates of sign-selective PPn neurons (bottom panels) as a function of the magnitude of the Df between the jamming signal and the fish's own signal. Each column represents data from one individual fish. Different symbols represent different neurons. Solid lines in bottom panels connect data for negative Dfs, broken lines connect data for positive Dfs. Note correspondence between behavioral and neuronal tuning curves for each individual. (From Rose et al. 1988)

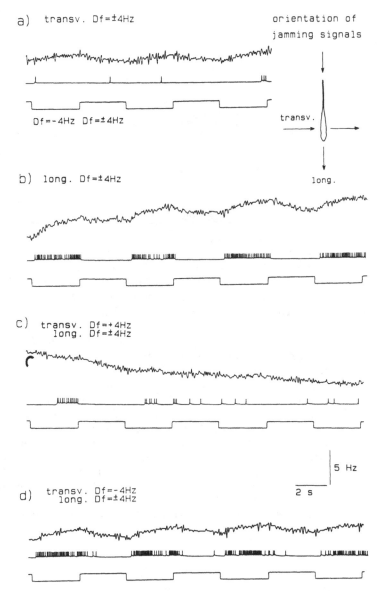

Figure 4.46
Nonlinear interaction between jamming signals that were delivered
through orthogonal pairs of electrodes (inset, upper right). This particular
PPn neuron showed unusual dependence upon the orientation of the jamming signal and almost failed to respond for the transverse orientation (*a*,
presentation of data as in figure 4.42*a*), while responding vigorously for the
longitudinal orientation (*b*). With a positive Df maintained for the transverse orientation, however, behavioral and neuronal responses to the
switching sign of the Df in the longitudinal field were largely suppressed
(*c*). No such interference was seen when the Df in the transverse field was
constantly negative (*d*). (From Rose et al. 1988)

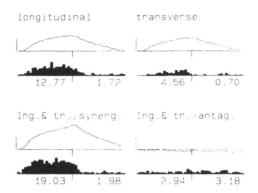

Figure 4.47
Synergistic and antagonistic effects of a longitudinally and a transversely
oriented jamming signal on recruitment of sign-selective PPn neuron. As
in figure 4.46, both signals had a magnitude of Df of 4 Hz, but both changed
their sign of Df synchronously every 2.3 s. Each panel is arranged as in
figure 4.41*b*, with the scale bar for the JAR being 1 Hz. The left halves of
the histograms cover the period of stimulation with the negative Df, and
the right halves of the histograms cover the subsequent period of stimulation with the positive Df. The numbers underneath give the respective
spike rates per second, calculated from the sixth bin to the last bin in each
half of the histogram. The sign of Df switches at the vertical tick mark
from negative to positive. Under synergistic stimulation (lower left panel),
the signs of the two Dfs were always identical, leading approximately to
an addition of the responses obtained for longitudinal and transverse stimulation alone (top panels). Under antagonistic stimulation (lower right
panel), the signs of the two Dfs were always opposite. Behavioral and
neuronal responses ceased under this condition, and the rate of firing of
the neuron was indistinguishable from that in the absence of any jamming.
Each panel contains data averaged over 11 to 19 modulation cycles of the
sign of Df. (From Rose et al. 1988)

the PPn, and if neurons of the nE that are excited by negative Dfs formed excitatory synapses on the distal portions of the same dendrites.

THE MEDULLARY PACEMAKER NUCLEUS: CONTROL OF THE ELECTRIC ORGAN

The medullary pacemaker of gymnotiform electric fish contains two classes of neurons, *pacemaker cells* and *relay cells*. The pacemaker cells are electrotonically coupled, fire synchronously, and drive the relay cells, which transmit each pacemaker command pulse to the spinal motor neurons of the electric organ (see figure 3.1) (Bennett 1971, and more recent review by Dye and Meyer 1986). Therefore, each EOD cycle is elicited by a single command pulse from the pacemaker nucleus. The activity of the pacemaker is modulated by inputs from neurons of the prepacemaker nucleus, which form synapses on pacemaker cells as well as relay cells (Szabo et al. 1989).

Gymnotiform fish with wave-type EODs, such as *Eigenmannia* and *Apteronotus*, normally generate EOD cycles of extreme regularity. The length of successive EOD intervals of an isolated, undisturbed fish, resting in water of constant temperature, may show a coefficient of variation (i.e., a standard deviation divided by the mean) as small as 0.0001. For an *Apteronotus* firing at 1000 Hz (i.e., with an EOD interval of 1 ms) this implies a standard deviation in the length of successive intervals as small as 0.1 μs (Bullock et al. 1975). The jitter produced by regular electronic function generators is not smaller, and the pacemakers of gymnotiform fish with wave-type EODs so far represent the most accurate biological oscillators.

The study of the medullary pacemaker has benefited from the fact that the pacemaker nucleus of the genus *Apteronotus* can be isolated in a brain slice preparation and maintained functional for days (Maler et al. 1983, Meyer 1984, Dye 1988). Most significantly, afferent fibers of the pacemaker can be saved in this preparation and stimulated electrically to generate both rapid, chirplike modulations and slowly decaying, JAR-like frequency elevations (Dye

and Heiligenberg 1987, Dye 1988). Since smooth, long-term frequency rises have a higher stimulation threshold than chirps, they
appear to be driven by thinner afferent fibers. This is in agreement
with the observation that stimulation of the small cells in the PPn-
G, which have thinner axons than the multipolar cells of the PPn-
C, generates similar smooth frequency rises of the pacemaker frequency. Simultaneous recording from pacemaker and relay cells
revealed that chirps are initiated in the relay cells and that the
pacemaker cells, which are coupled electrotonically to the relay
cells, then follow the firing pattern of the latter. This indicates that
the multipolar cells of the PPn-C, which drive chirps in the pacemaker, innervate the relay cells directly. On the other hand, smooth
frequency rises may originate from innervation of the pacemaker
cells by the small cells of the PPn-G. Ultrastructural studies of
labeled afferent axons of known origin are required to confirm these
assumptions. A very significant functional separation of pacemaker
and relay cell innervation has also been found in the related pulse-
type gymnotiform genus *Hypopomus* (Kawasaki and Heiligenberg
1989, 1990).

By in vivo as well as in vitro application of different pharmacological agents to the pacemaker of *Eigenmannia* and *Apteronotus*,
Dye et al. (1989) were able to show that prepacemaker modulation
of the EOD frequency was mediated by glutaminergic transmission
in the pacemaker nucleus. Moreover, the smooth frequency rises
appear to be mediated by NMDA (N-methyl-D-aspartate) receptors,
while chirps appear to be mediated by kainate/quisqualate receptors
(figure 4.48). While application of the NMDA blocker APV (D(−)2-
amino-5-phosphonovaleric acid), selectively and reversibly suppressed the JAR, application of the kainate/quisqualate blocker
GAMS (γ-D-glutamylamino-methylsulphonic acid), as well as the
more recently tested drug CNQX (6-cyano-7-nitroquinoxaline-2,3-
dione), selectively and reversibly attenuated chirps (figure 4.49). By
virtue of separate patterns of innervations and the employment of
different types of receptors, the pacemaker nucleus is thus capable
of executing very different forms of modulations simultaneously
and independently. An even richer variety of modulations has been

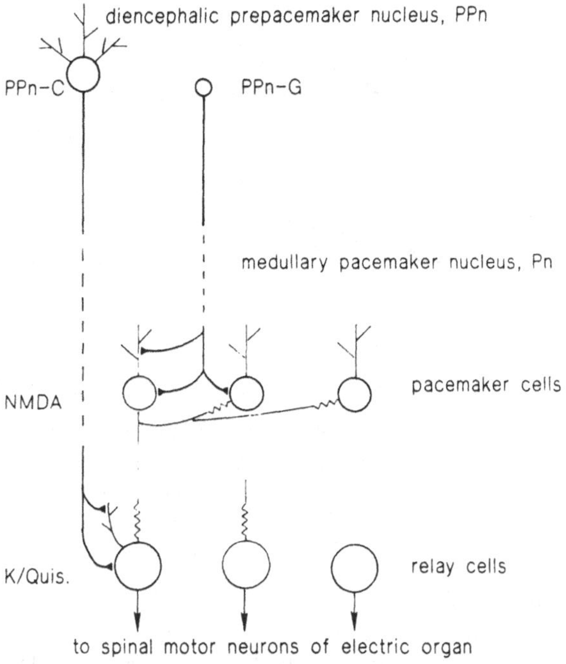

Figure 4.48
The diencephalic PPn consists of two subunits, the PPn-G and the PPn-C, and innervates the medullary pacemaker nucleus (Pn). While activation of the PPn-G causes a gradual rise of the pacemaker frequency, activation of the PPn-C causes "chirps," abrupt rises in frequency that may lead to a brief interruption of the pacemaker cycle. The pacemaker nucleus consists of electrotonically coupled pacemaker cells and relay cells. Although the synaptic targets of the PPn-G and PPn-C cannot yet be distinguished (Szabo et al. 1989), indirect evidence suggests that the PPn-C innervates the relay cells directly. Whereas NMDA receptors mediate smooth rises of the pacemaker frequency, kainate/quisqualate receptors mediate chirps (see figure 4.49).

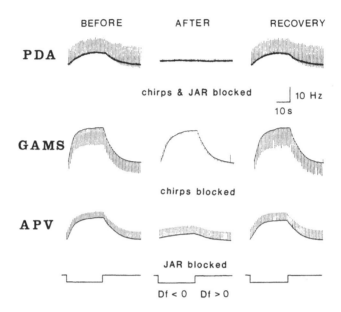

Figure 4.49
Under the control of the diencephalic PPn, the medullary pacemaker
nucleus can produce the gradual frequency modulations of the JAR as well
as the abrupt chirps used in courtship and aggression. Either form of modulation can selectively and reversibly be suppressed by injection of specific
glutamate receptor blockers into the pacemaker. A curarized *Eigenmannia*
was induced to perform a JAR (smooth modulations in pacemaker frequency records) by continually being exposed to a jamming signal which
was alternately 4 Hz lower (Df < 0) or 4 Hz higher (Df > 0) in frequency
(bottom trace) than its own EOD substitute signal. Simultaneously, an
electric stimulus pulse was delivered through a microelectrode to a population of neurons in the PPn once every second to generate a chirplike
frequency modulation (vertical pulses in pacemaker frequency records).
While the nonspecific glutamate blocker PDA blocked both responses (top
record), the kainate/quisqualate blocker GAMS blocked only chirping (center record), and the NMDA blocker APV only suppressed the JAR (bottom
record). Recovery from these treatments occurred within a few minutes.
Representative records are shown in this figure, with different individuals
chosen for each type of drug application. Chirps are brief and sudden rises
in pacemaker frequency which, depending on the intensity and location of
the electric stimulus being applied to the PPn, may proceed without a
significant attenuation of the pacemaker signal (pulses pointing upward
from trace of sustained pacemaker frequency), or may lead to an attenuation
so strong that the pacemaker cycle appears to be interrupted, thus causing
a momentary drop in apparent pacemaker frequency (pulses pointing downward from trace of sustained pacemaker frequency). (From Dye et al. 1989)

documented in the pulse-species *Hypopomus* (Kawasaki and Heiligenberg 1989, 1990).

A SUMMARY FLOW DIAGRAM OF NEURONAL STRUCTURES AND FUNCTIONS CONTROLLING THE JAR

The neuronal pathway controlling the JAR is set out in figure 4.50, and the form of coding of information by different classes of neurons is outlined schematically in figure 4.51. Phase and amplitude information are coded by T-type and P-type receptors, respectively, and are processed separately within the ELL of the hindbrain (figure 4.52). The JAR requires that the animal recognize local rises and falls in stimulus amplitude in relation to the differential phase of the stimulus with respect to a reference signal monitored at some other point of the body surface. Local rises and falls in stimulus amplitude are detected within the ELL, while differential phase is computed within lamina 6 of the torus semicircularis of the midbrain. Amplitude and differential phase information converge in deeper laminae of the torus where sign-selective cells recognize particular combinations of phase and amplitude modulations which in total reflect the sign of the Df between the neighbor's jamming signal and the animal's own EOD. Information about the sign of Df provided by these cells is still ambiguous, however, whereas higher-order, sign-selective cells in the nE code the sign of Df more reliably. The nE also shows distinct premotor areas, nE↑ and nE↓, which are necessary for the JAR by controlling rises and falls in EOD frequency, respectively. The nE, in turn, innervates the area of the PPn that contains highly sign-selective neurons in the subnucleus PPn-G. These neurons are excited by negative Dfs, which cause a rise in EOD frequency, and are inhibited by positive Dfs, which cause a fall in EOD frequency. These neurons innervate the medullary pacemaker, which drives each EOD cycle by a single command pulse, and modulate its frequency smoothly and continually.

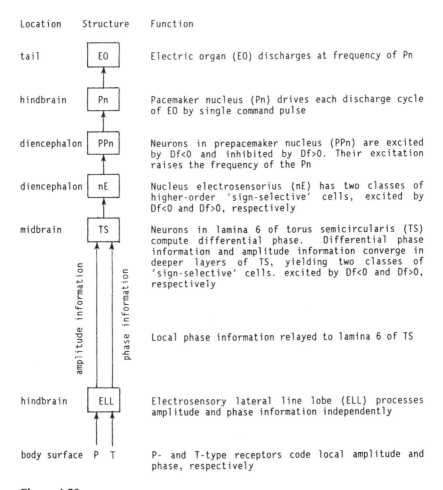

Figure 4.50
A flow diagram of neuronal structures and their functions in the context
of the JAR. This diagram only contains elements whose significance for
the JAR has been demonstrated experimentally. Details of the coding of
sensory information are shown schematically in figure 4.51. The interconnections of all known electrosensory structures are mapped in the diagram
of figure 4.52.

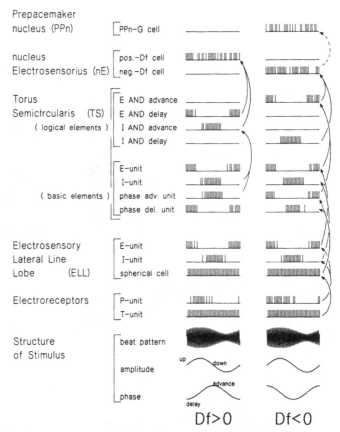

Figure 4.51
The sign of the Df between the neighbor's EOD and the fish's own is coded along a succession of central nervous stations outlined in figure 4.50. The structure of the beat patterns for positive and negative Dfs is shown at the bottom, and the form of their phase modulations is derived from a comparison of these beat patterns with representations of the fish's own EOD less strongly contaminated by the neighbor's signal. Curved arrows to the right of symbolic spike records indicate the flow of information among the classes of neurons involved. To minimize clutter, only some connections have been indicated between the "basic elements" and "logical elements" of the torus. The assumed structure of the logical elements, also referred to as "sign-selective" cells, has been discussed in connection with figure 4.31. The use of the AND operation should not imply strict and-gating as in electronic circuits but rather indicate a general form of nonlinear facilitation between an amplitude-coding input (E- or I-type) and a phase-coding input (phase advance-coding unit or phase delay-coding unit). The nature of the connections from torus to nE is still unknown, and the arrows should only indicate a possible way of wiring. Also unknown are the connections from the nE to the prepacemaker nucleus, a subnucleus (PPn-G) of which contains cells inhibited by positive Dfs and excited by negative Dfs. The activation of these cells, in turn, raises the frequency of the medullary pacemaker.

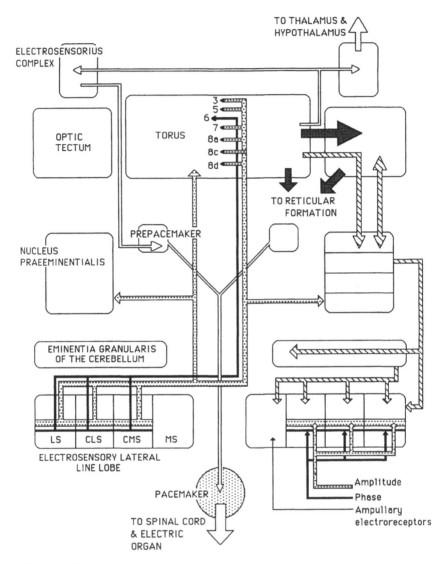

Figure 4.52
Electrosensory structures and their interconnections in *Eigenmannia*. For the sake of clarity, many connections have been drawn only unilaterally. The four segments of the ELL are the medial (MS), centromedial (CMS), centrolateral (CLS), and lateral (LS) segments. Other details of the recurrent connections between the nucleus praeeminentialis and the ELL are given in figure 4.16. (Courtesy of C.E. Carr)

5   General Principles in the Neuronal Organization of the Jamming Avoidance Response

Although the electric sense may appear to be an unusual modality, a comparison with other sensory systems reveals that its neuronal organization follows very similar principles. Whenever sensory information of any kind is represented in ordered neuronal maps, very general rules can be applied for the extraction of specific stimulus features and for the subsequent conversion of sensory codes into motor programs. Such rules and their presence in different systems will be considered in the following. Many of these points have been discussed in recent reviews (Heiligenberg 1991; Konishi 1991).

THE SEPARATION OF TASK-SPECIFIC SENSORY CHANNELS

The perceptual machinery of a given animal species is tuned to sensory modalities and stimulus variables that are essential for the control of its behavioral repertoire. Behavioral experiments in ants and bees have identified various types of photoreceptors that differ in their spectral sensitivities and serve separate behavioral functions. Photoreceptors sensitive to the plane of polarization of ultraviolet light control navigation with reference to the polarization pattern of the blue sky (Wehner 1989a,b), whereas green-sensitive photoreceptors serve in the discrimination of visual contours and their motion (Lehrer and Srinivasan 1989, Lehrer et al. 1990, Srinivasan et al. 1990). In a similar manner, ampullary electroreceptors of gymnotiform and mormyriform fishes are sensitive to low-frequency signals of various geophysical and biophysical origins, while tuberous electroreceptors in the same species are tuned to the high spectral frequencies of its electric organ discharges that serve in social communication and the electrolocation of moving objects (see chapter 2).

This behavioral specialization of receptor types at the periphery is reflected by distinct central representations of their inputs and largely independent mechanisms for the early processing of their information. The ampullary and tuberous electroreceptors, which are distributed over the body surface of gymnotiform and mormyriform fishes, project to separate, somatotopically ordered maps in the electrosensory lateral line lobe (ELL, see chapter 4) of the hindbrain. Moreover, the tuberous receptors of gymnotiform fish fall into two classes, T-units and P-units, which are adapted to code the phase and the amplitude of periodic electric signals, respectively. And these two classes of tuberous receptors project to different higher-order cell populations that segregate processing of phase and amplitude information. A similar central separation of phase and amplitude information is seen in the auditory system of the barn owl (Konishi et al. 1988, Takahashi 1989). But here, the two pathways do not start with different types of receptors at the periphery. Instead, each auditory receptor projects to two targets in the brainstem, the nucleus magnocellularis and the nucleus angularis, which extract phase and amplitude information, respectively, and form the beginning of two pathways that follow separate routes up to the level of the midbrain.

A similar, although more complex separation of channels is found in the primate visual system. Two classes of retinal ganglion cells compute information provided by the rods and cones in different ways. They generate two visual systems, magnocellular and parvocellular, which differ in their spatial and temporal acuity as well as in their discrimination of colors, follow distinct routes to separate cortical representations, and serve different visual tasks (Livingstone and Hubel 1987, DeYoe and van Essen 1988). A similar tradeoff between temporal and spatial acuity is seen in the electrosensory system of gymnotiform fish. Each tuberous electroreceptor afferent projects to three separate somatotopically organized maps in the ELL of the hindbrain (see chapter 4), which serves in the analysis of electric images on the animal's body surface. Although these three maps lack conspicuous qualitative differences, their higher-order neurons differ in their spatial and temporal response properties. A comparison of neurons in the most lateral and the most medial map reveals that those in the lateral map show higher temporal acuity and those in the most medial map show higher spatial acuity. Neurons in a third map, located between these two, show intermediate properties (Shumway 1989a,b). This example strongly supports the original proposal by Allman and Kaas (1971, 1974) and Allman et al. (1981) that new maps emerge through reduplication of established maps and then follow separate paths of specialization. The apparently subtle differences seen in the three maps of the electrosensory system suggest that these maps emerged recently in evolutionary time and may still undergo further differentiation.

Separate substrates and pathways probably evolved whenever different forms of information required more accurate coding and could no longer be processed within the same neural network. The background noise of individual elements within a sensory map limits their ability to code rapid modulations of their input signal. The pooled information obtained from a sufficiently large population of such elements will improve temporal acuity, but this pooling will also entail a loss in spatial acuity. Separate structures should thus evolve for enhanced temporal and spatial representations. A network analyzing the phase (i.e., the timing of the zero-crossing of a sinusoidal electric or auditory signal), may be required to operate with very different signal amplitudes and to tolerate fluctuations in amplitude without significant distortions in the coding of phase. This operation calls for a synaptic organization very different from that in a system designed for the coding of signal amplitude. Separate substrates may evolve in the form of distinct nuclei, as in the case of the cochlear nuclei of the owl, or in the form of different laminae within the same structure, as in the case of the electrosensory lateral line lobe and torus semicircularis of gymnotiform fish.

THE CENTRAL CONVERGENCE OF CHANNELS AND THE CONVERSION
OF NEURONAL CODES

The initial segregation of stimulus variables, such as phase and amplitude in the auditory system of owls or the electrosensory system of fish, is followed by a convergence of their data flows at still higher centers which serve in the recognition of particular patterns formed by these variables. Barn owls determine the azimuth and elevation of an auditory target on the basis of interaural differences in phase and amplitude, respectively, and "space-specific" neurons in the inferior colliculus respond to the combination of these variables and form an ordered map of auditory space (Konishi et al. 1988, Takahashi 1989). The gymnotiform electric fish, *Eigenmannia*, recognizes the sign of a frequency difference between a neighbor's signal and its own signal by analyzing modulations in the phase and amplitude of the interference pattern formed by the mixing of the two signals (see chapter 3). Higher-order electrosensory neurons execute the necessary joint evaluation of phase and amplitude information within the torus semicircularis where the pathways carrying these two forms of information converge (see chapter 4, The Gating of Amplitude Information by Phase Information).

The convergence of pathways and the emergence of higher-order neurons may be accompanied by a change in their neuronal codes, and the extraction and coding of particular aspects of a stimulus pattern commonly involves the gradual rejection of other stimulus features. In gymnotiform fish, T-type receptor afferents mark the timing of the zero-crossing, or phase, of a sinusoidal signal by firing a single spike at a fixed latency within each cycle of the signal. This information is coded for many points on the body surface, and it is relayed in the same form and in somatotopic register, by the spherical cells of the electrosensory lateral line lobe, to lamina 6 of the torus semicircularis in the midbrain (see chapter 4). A network within lamina 6 compares the arrival times of spikes from pairs of regions on the body surface, and small cells at a location in lamina 6 representing a given region A on the body surface modulate their rate of firing in accordance with the difference between the timing of the signal in A and some other area, B. The firing of these small cells is irregular and no longer locked to individual cycles of the sinusoidal signal. In one type of small cell, the firing rate increases if region A experiences a small phase lead with respect to region B, and it decreases below its resting level if A experiences a small phase lag. The modulation in firing rate of small cells located at the somatotopic representation of region A in lamina 6 codes only the differential phase of the signal in region A with reference to some other region, while information about the exact timing of signals in any individual region is discarded at this level.

The auditory system of the barn owl shows a tonotopic organization in the phase-coding and amplitude-coding pathways up to the level of the inferior colliculus. At this point, an apparent convergence of neurons tuned to different frequencies but identical interaural temporal disparities yields an array of higher-order units that no longer discriminate frequencies and only respond to specific azimuth angles of a sound source. The ordered spatial arrangement of these units according to the angle of their preferred azimuth of sound origin then yields a neuronal map of azimuthal space (Konishi et al. 1988, Takahashi 1989).

More complex forms of neuronal representations of behaviorally relevant features, or "information-bearing parameters" (Suga 1984, 1988a,b), have been found in the auditory cortex of bats. In some cases, the original tonotopic organization is abandoned, and other aspects of auditory information are coded instead. The echolocation sounds of bats consist of constant frequency (CF) components and frequency-modulated (FM) components, which are adapted to specific tasks in target detection and evaluation. Whereas CF sounds are optimal for the detection of faint echoes, measurement of relative flight speed, and evaluation of an insect's wingbeat rate, FM sounds are more suitable for the discrimination of target distance and texture. Simmons (1973) predicted that species with echolocation sounds dominated by an FM component should show better target range discrimination than species with relatively longer CF components. When he found that both types performed equally well, he proposed that bats might process CF and FM components separately and assess different aspects of sonar information in parallel. The presence of a long CF component would thus not impair the assessment of target range by selective use of the FM component. This postulate was supported by Suga's discovery (Suga 1988a) that CF and FM information are indeed represented in different portions of the auditory cortex. In the mustached bat, *Pteronotus*, for example, one finds a Doppler-shifted CF (DSCF) processing area with an ordered mapping of the frequency and the amplitude of CF sounds, and an FM-FM area, which forms a map of target distance by an arrangement of neurons tuned to progressively shorter temporal separations between the fundamental FM component of the outgoing echolocation sound and specific higher-harmonic FM components of the returning echo. Different aspects of biologically relevant sonar information are thus represented in separate neuronal maps.

THE REPRESENTATION OF STIMULUS VARIABLES IN ORDERED MAPS

Wherever one finds behavioral responses guided by continual modulations of a certain stimulus variable, an ordered representation of this variable within neuronal maps is generally found as well. Whereas the existence of retinotopic, somatotopic, or tonotopic maps could be interpreted as a developmental consequence of topographic projections of sensory surfaces, other maps are constructed and ordered by computations (Konishi 1986). The inferior colliculus of owls contains an ordered representation of auditory space based on the joint computation of interaural differences in phase and amplitude (Konishi et al. 1988, Takahashi 1989), and this map obviously forms a neuronal substrate for the tracking of auditory targets. To the extent that the flow of either phase or amplitude information to this map is impaired, neurons there show losses in the acuity of their spatial tuning, and tracking performance of the head suffers similarly. The pursuit of a flying insect by the bat *Pteronotus* is controlled by changes in target distance, which is mapped continually within the FM-FM area of its auditory cortex on the basis of echo delay measurements (Suga 1988a).

All sensory maps known in gymnotiform electric fish are ordered somatotopically and serve in the spatial analysis of perturbations in the electric events on the fish's body surface. Such perturbations are caused by the motion of nearby objects (see figures 2.2, 2.3) as well by the interference with electric organ discharges (EODs) of neighbors (figure 3.4). The detection of the direction of motion requires comparisons of changes in transepidermal signals between neighboring receptive fields, much as light levels must be compared across neighboring points on a retina for the detection of visual motion (Borst and Egelhaaf 1989). The assessment of a neighbor's EOD interfering with the fish's own EOD requires comparisons of amplitude and phase information sampled at different locations on the body surface, and rather large receptive fields might suffice in the case of the JAR (see figure 4.33). Whereas the necessary phase comparisons are computed in lamina 6 of the torus, the joint spatial computation of phase and amplitude information is facilitated by the topographic alignment of lamina 6 with amplitude-coding laminae above and below (see chapter 4). Vertical connections between these laminae thus achieve a matching of spatially congruent phase and amplitude information.

The somatotopic order of electrosensory information is abandoned beyond the level of the torus semicircularis and tectum opticum. The torus, which performs spatial computations of electrosensory information necessary for the JAR, projects to the nucleus electrosensorius (nE). This diencephalic nucleus lacks a somatotopic organization and instead contains a motor map in the form of two subnuclei, nE↑ and nE↓, which govern the motor output of the JAR by raising and lowering the pacemaker frequency, respectively (see chapter 4). Similarly, the electrosensory map within the tectum is also organized somatotopically, and its spatial register with a visual map of the fish's environment gives rise to multimodal neurons responding to various qualities of moving objects (Bastian 1982, 1986a, Heiligenberg and Rose 1987). Here, a deep layer of tectal neurons projecting to higher-order structures reveals a motor-map organization in the form of a topographic representation of swimming direction (Yuthas 1985), reminding us of a similar representation of eye-movement vectors in the superior colliculus of primates (Sparks 1986, 1988, 1989; Sparks and Mays 1990).

One can imagine a variety of advantages that ordered representations in neuronal maps might offer. If the quantity of a stimulus variable is coded by the location of the map being excited, and if this location varies continuously with a gradual variation of this quantity, then temporal variations of this quantity should cause motions of the excited locus within this map. Such motions could be detected by a general network structure similar to that employed for visual motion detection in a retina or compound eye. The ontogenetic organization of such networks could follow simple rules defining connections as a function of relative distance and position of elements within the matrix of neurons. In a scrambled map, however, every individual connection would require a specific instruction, and a table of such instructions could easily exhaust the volume of available genetic information.

A further advantage of an ordered representation appears to be that it offers the potential for enhanced acuity and, ultimately, hyperacuity. Neurons in the FM-FM area of the auditory cortex of the mustached bat, *Pteronotus*, are tuned rather broadly to specific ranges of target distance. On the basis of the density of the spacing of FM-FM neurons within this map, one can calculate that the best echo delay times between neighbors differ by 0.13 ms. However, behavioral tests of target distance discrimination show that the bat is capable of detecting differences as small as 1 to 1.5 cm, which correspond to a difference in the associated echo delay times of 0.06 to 0.09 ms (Simmons 1973). This acuity is approximately twice as high as expected from the resolution of the FM-FM area (Suga and Horikawa 1986). Even larger discrepancies are seen between our visual vernier acuity and the spacing of photoreceptors in the retina (Westheimer and McKee 1977). Theoretical considerations show that a form of weighted averaging of inputs from neighboring elements within a map of broadly tuned neurons can yield a degree of acuity of perception which far exceeds that expected from the coarseness of the map and that acuity is, within limits, enhanced by the broadening of the tuning. Moreover, very simple and robust rules can be proposed for the ontogeny of the necessary wiring of such maps (Heiligenberg 1987, 1989; Baldi and Heiligenberg 1988). As a natural consequence, the ordered representation of a sensory space by broadly tuned neurons also offers a distributed coding of motor outputs if the length and direction of vectors characterizing movements in space are mapped continually and in topographic register with the sensory representation. Eye movements in primates represent an example (Sparks 1986, 1988, 1989; Choongkil et al. 1988). They appear to be generated by the recruitment of a local population of broadly tuned neurons within an ordered motor map of the superior colliculus. The location of the center of this population determines the direction and magnitude of the movement, and a bell-shaped weight function defines the strength of recruitment in the vicinity of this center. It remains to be tested whether a similar spatial weighting principle also holds for the control of hand movements by weighted recruitment of units within a population of directionally tuned cortical neurons (Georgopoulos et al. 1988, 1989).

Laminated and topographically ordered strata of neurons thus appear well adapted for the processing of sensory information for several reasons, and it therefore surprises us that core regions in the ectostriatum of the avian telencephalon may perform complex computations of ordered spatial information without being laminated (Karten and Shimizu 1990). Detailed physiological and anatomical studies of these structures should teach us much about the computational constraints of laminated and nonlaminated neuronal substrates.

THE EMERGENCE OF "RECOGNITION" NEURONS AND MOTOR PROGRAMS

Perceptual neurons of sufficiently high order may respond very selectively to a specific, biologically relevant stimulus pattern (Ewert 1987, Perrett et al. 1989, Schildberger 1989). A comparison of neurons at different hierarchical levels shows that this selectivity emerges gradually as one ascends to higher levels. The gymnotiform electric fish, *Eigenmannia*, for example, recognizes the sign of the frequency difference (Df) between a neighbor's signal and its own signal and controls shifts of its pacemaker frequency accordingly. This jamming avoidance response (JAR) occurs independently of the spatial orientation of the neighbor's signal, and a fish may readily detect signals more than a thousand times weaker than its own. Neurons that reliably code the sign of Df, regardless of the orientation of the neighbor's signal, and with a sensitivity comparable to that observed at the behavioral level, are found in the prepacemaker nucleus of the diencephalon (see chapter 4). The neurons of this nucleus are at least seven synaptic levels from the electroreceptors on the body surface, and they modulate the firing frequency of the medullary pacemaker nucleus, which drives the electric organ and thereby determines the fish's own signal frequency. The responses of afferent neurons of sufficiently low order, such as those in the torus semicircularis of the midbrain, depend on the orientation of the neighbor's signal, and while a neuron may prefer a positive Df for one orientation it may prefer a negative Df for another. Moreover, these lower-order neurons are far less sensitive to weak signals, and their discrimination of the sign of Df can therefore only be demonstrated by averaging their responses over periods of time much longer than required for the behavioral response (Rose and Heiligenberg 1986a,b). In addition, the firing rate of these neurons is strongly modulated by the temporal beat pattern formed by the interference of the animal's own signal with that of its neighbor, while the neurons of the prepacemaker nucleus fire at a rather even rate, which is elevated for negative Dfs, when the animal raises its own frequency, and suppressed for positive Dfs, when the animal lowers its frequency (see figure 4.41). The responses of these high-order neurons thus perfectly reflect the stimulus selectivity and dynamic properties of the JAR and are immune to behaviorally irrelevant stimulus features.

The high sensitivity and coding fidelity of the prepacemaker neurons can be explained through convergence of information flow from lower-order neurons in the torus semicircularis via the diencephalic nucleus electrosensorius (Keller 1988, Keller and Heiligen-berg 1989, Keller et al. 1990). Whereas individual neurons of lower order do not code the sign of Df reliably, one can show that the pooling of responses of a large set of such neurons will always yield an unambiguous representation of the sign of Df (Heiligenberg and Rose 1986). In addition, such pooling will also achieve a higher sensitivity to weak interfering signals. As mentioned above, sign-selective responses to sufficiently weak signals can only be dem-onstrated after extensive averaging over time. Parallel convergence of the responses of such neurons, however, should yield a discrim-ination of the sign of Df with a latency as short as that observed at the behavioral level. The highest-order neurons may thus display a sensitivity comparable to that at the behavioral level and orders of magnitude better than that of individual receptors (Kawasaki et al. 1988b).

The neurons in the prepacemaker nucleus of gymnotiform fish not only represent an advanced level of a neuronal hierarchy pro-cessing sensory information, they also participate in a motor path-way controlling the firing of the electric organ in response to the stimulus patterns that they perceive. The prepacemaker nucleus contains two sets of cells, both of which project to the pacemaker nucleus: a cluster of small, ovoid cells and an assembly of larger, multipolar cells. The small cells, which were described above, dis-criminate the sign of Df in a JAR. They fire spontaneously and are excited by a small negative Df (i.e., when the neighbor's signal is of lower frequency), and they are inhibited by a small positive Df. Since excitation of the small cells raises the pacemaker frequency, a fish raises its signal frequency for a negative Df and lowers its frequency for a positive Df. This causal link can be demonstrated by stimulating these small cells with iontophoretic applications of L-glutamate (Kawasaki et al. 1988a). Activation of the large cells, on the other hand, causes rapid modulations in the pacemaker frequency, as they are naturally observed in the context of aggres-sion and courtship in a behavior called chirping. Depolarization of a single large cell can induce at least a weak form of chirping, whereas stronger chirps presumably require the joint recruitment

of many neurons of this type. And while the activation of a single
neuron suffices to trigger a chirp, this particular neuron does not
necessarily participate in the generation of every chirp (Kawasaki
et al. 1988a). In this regard, prepacemaker neurons very much
resemble the classic command neurons of crayfish; they are sufficient to drive the behavior but not individually necessary (Larimer
1988).

The gradual frequency modulations of the JAR and the chirplike
modulations expressed during courtship and aggression are generated within the same network of the medullary pacemaker nucleus
(see chapter 4). Pharmacological manipulations indicate that gradual frequency modulations are mediated by NMDA receptors,
whereas chirps are elicited via kainate/quisqualate receptors (Dye
et al. 1989). The same network of cells in the medullary pacemaker
can thus be modulated in different ways to generate distinct forms
of electric organ activity. Early ethology postulated a local representation of motor patterns, and this notion was supported by brain
stimulation experiments which identified diencephalic regions that
appeared to trigger complex, natural forms of behavior. The studies
on the electrosensory system, which have addressed this issue at
the single-cell level, similarly show that a local neuronal representation of behavioral patterns can only be observed at the level of
the diencephalic prepacemaker nucleus, whereas a distributed and
overlapping network of motor elements is utilized in the medullary
pacemaker nucleus to generate different forms of behavior. Much
as we see a convergence, or fanning-in, of pathways toward the
prepacemaker nucleus from the sensory side, we observe a diver-
gence, or fanning-out, of pathways from sensory structures towards
motor elements.

The modulation of a neuronal circuitry for the generation of
different motor patterns has been established through studies of
rhythm-generating systems in invertebrates (Getting 1989a, Katz
and Harris-Warrick 1990, Harris-Warrick and Marder 1991) as well
as vertebrates (Bekoff 1986; Bekoff et al. 1987, 1989; Stein et al.
1986; Grillner et al. 1988). The effects of afferent inputs range from
the subtle modulations of a motor pattern observed in the stabili-

zation of locust flight (Rowell 1989) to the switching between different patterns of coordination in the mollusc, *Tritonia* (Getting 1989b). And the state of a motor circuit, in turn, may weigh or gate the effects of afferent inputs (Hoy et al. 1989).

THE DISTRIBUTED PROCESSING OF SENSORY INFORMATION AND THE SHARED USE OF NEURONAL CIRCUITS

The neuronal system governing the JAR lacks particular, singular neurons that exercise a pivotal function and therefore are indispensable. No single neuron has been identified so far that might be considered a main controller or governor of this behavior; instead, whole classes of neurons fulfill certain functions. As a consequence, the system is resistant to physical trauma. The JAR survives the loss of large areas of body surface as well as extensive lesions within the ELL and torus semicircularis. The only behavioral impairment is an eventual reduction of the size of the frequency shifts elicited by a given jamming regimen and a loss of sensitivity to very weak interfering signals. Since the detection of weak interfering signals requires that information from a large population of receptors and higher-order neurons be pooled (Kawasaki et al. 1988b), sensitivity to weak signals degrades with progressive loss of sensory elements.

Much as we see a sharing of neuronal structures at the motor level for the generation of different behavioral responses (as discussed earlier), we also find a sharing of structures for the analysis of sensory information in different behavioral contexts. Several types of neurons in the torus are driven by amplitude and phase modulations, regardless of whether these are generated by interference of the fish's own EOD with that of a neighbor or by an object moving in the vicinity, and responses to moving objects may easily be masked by responses to interference patterns (Rose et al. 1987). Since such neurons project to the tectum as well as to the nE (see chapter 4), their information can be processed for motion analysis within the tectum and for the assessment of social signals within the nE. A further subdivision of the nE then yields two subnuclei, the nE↑ and nE↓, for control of the JAR, and two more subnuclei, the nEb and nEar, apparently for the processing of electric signals in the context of aggression and courtship (Heiligenberg et al. 1991).

The JAR of *Eigenmannia* is driven most strongly by frequency differences (Df) of a magnitude in the range from 2 to 6 Hz between interfering signals (see chapter 3). Chirping responses, on the other hand, can be elicited over a much wider range of Dfs. In the related genus *Apteronotus*, magnitudes of Df between 9 and 16 Hz are most effective in eliciting chirps, whereas values between 1 and 6 Hz are most effective for the JAR (Dye 1987). Neurons of the torus vary widely in their ranges of Df that are optimal for their recruitment, although neurons tuned to Dfs most effective for the JAR form a majority (Partridge et al. 1981). Many toral neurons could contribute to the JAR as well as to the chirp response, and statistical differences in their projections dependent upon their Df-tuning would suffice to bring about the differences in the Df-tuning of the JAR and chirping.

THE CONTROL OF MOTIVATIONAL STATES THROUGH SOCIAL SIGNALS

A principal function of social communication is to allow animals to manipulate the behavioral state of their partners by continual emission of stereotyped signals. Lehrman (1965) and his collaborators demonstrated the significance of courtship signals for the induction of ovulation in doves and lizards (Crews 1975); Wingfield (1985) observed changes in hormonal titers as a function of the outcome of social encounters in birds (Wingfield and Moore 1987, Wingfield and Marler 1988). The exposure to specific social signals changes certain states of behavioral readiness in animals as diverse as fish and insects, and these effects dissipate exponentially with time constants ranging from seconds to days, depending on the particular stimulus pattern and type of behavior involved (Heiligenberg 1977b). It appears plausible that the perception of a specific stimulus causes a sudden rise in the level of some modulatory substance and that the following diffusion or destruction of this substance leads to an exponential decay of the behavioral effect.

Little is known about neuronal structures that detect social signals and then initiate changes in the hormonal state of the animal. In the context of aggression and courtship, the gymnotiform electric fish, *Eigenmannia*, repeatedly and briefly interrupts its normally continuous electric organ discharges by chirping. This signal is produced most frequently during the hours of spawning, and females will only release their eggs in response to long sequences of chirping produced by a male in close proximity. This signal is so effective that sufficiently gravid females, after removal of all males, will spawn in the vicinity of electrodes through which a male's chirping is played back into the water (Hagedorn 1986). Electrosensory neurons that respond to chirps form a pathway that leads through the torus semicircularis of the midbrain to a section of the nucleus electrosensorius, the nEar, and the lateral pretectum, both part of the diencephalon, and diencephalic neurons sensitive to chirping project to hypothalamic targets (Keller et al. 1989, 1990; Heiligenberg et al. 1991), which in turn may be linked to the pituitary (Johnston and Maler 1989). Along this pathway, a male's chirping might indeed manipulate the hormonal state of the female.

RECURRENT DESCENDING LOOPS: SEARCHLIGHTS AND CENTRAL REPRESENTATIONS OF SENSORY EXPECTATION?

The description of sensory processing presented so far has paid little attention to the existence of recurrent pathways (see chapter 4) and given the impression of a linear neuronal hierarchy leading to a motor output. Although descending recurrent projections are very common, little has been learned so far about their functional significance. Studies on the anatomy and physiology of a major recurrent loop in the electrosensory system of gymnotiform fish have revealed two separate functions, a general gain control affecting an entire stratum of neurons and a local effect limited to a small portion of this stratum. The ELL, which processes electric images, projects topographically to the nucleus praeeminentialis of the midbrain. This nucleus, in turn, projects back to the ELL, indirectly and diffusely via the lobus caudalis of the cerebellum, as well as directly and topographically (see figures 3.1, 4.16). The multipolar cells of the nucleus praeeminentialis project to the lobus caudalis, whose granule cells send a parallel fiber system through the dorsal dendrites of the pyramidal cells of the ELL. Reversible interruption of this recurrent pathway has shown that the pyramidal cells lose their ability to adapt to changes in overall stimulus amplitude and can no longer code electric images over a wide range of stimulus amplitude (Bastian 1986 a,b; Bastian and Bratton 1990). A degradation of vision under varying light levels would be a comparable situation. The stellate cells of the nucleus praeeminentialis, on the other hand, project directly back to the electrosensory lateral line lobe and form small terminal fields among the dendrites of the pyramidal cells (Maler et al. 1982, Bratton and Bastian 1990). This recurrent pathway, which appears to affect only small, local populations of cells, could selectively alter their response properties and play the role of an attention mechanism or "searchlight" (Crick 1984). Selective elimination or alteration of this feedback loop and studies of the ensuing behavioral and physiological consequences are needed to test this hypothesis.

A further function of descending loops might be to compare incoming information with patterns expected on the basis of previously gathered information. Bell (1989) has demonstrated that mormyriform electric fish use a corollary discharge signal of their electric organ discharge command to identify electrosensory feedback caused by their own discharges and to establish a continually updated internal representation of most recently obtained patterns of electrosensory information. This representation could be essential for the detection of novelties in the stream of afferent information. Bastian (personal communication) suggests a similar function for the descending pathway in gymnotiform fish.

DEVELOPMENTAL AND EVOLUTIONARY CONSIDERATIONS

Physiological and anatomical studies of neuronal structures always provoke questions regarding their developmental organization and evolutionary history. A neuronal network suggested to explain a specific function will appear plausible to the extent that it could develop on the basis of simple and robust rules governing the establishment of its connections. Developmental mechanisms certainly restrict the nature and the degree of structural complexity that neural networks can achieve and set boundaries for the course of their evolution. Moreover, new structures can only evolve by gradual modifications of existing designs and to the extent that their operation is compatible with existing adaptations that need to be maintained. Much as many other structural and functional features in organisms, neuronal designs reflect their evolutionary history (Dumont and Robertson 1986), and some even appear to be burdened by it. A number of specific neuronal solutions to problems of sensory information processing found in the electrosensory nervous system of certain fishes appear awkward, show traces of patchwork improvisations, and reveal the lack of long-range, goal-oriented planning (Heiligenberg 1987, 1989).

A striking example for a patchwork of improvements is seen in a correction of timing errors in the phase-comparing system of *Eigenmannia* discussed in connection with figure 4.34. Corrections are found at three levels. First, the fish has minimized temporal delays in the relaying of phase information from distant points of the body surface by increasing conduction speed in primary T-type afferents originating more distantly. This compensation, however, is far from perfect, and the arrival of action potentials originating from the caudal end of the trunk may still be delayed by almost 1 ms. This appears intolerable for a system that can resolve phase differences of less than 1 μs, and a second improvement in the analysis of phase differences is achieved at the level of the torus. Within lamina 6, phase comparisons are executed most abundantly between neighboring receptive fields, where differences in conduction delays of T-signals are minimal. A third correction is achieved at the next higher level. Phase-coding neurons in deeper laminae of the torus do not respond exclusively to the steady-state value of a phase difference but also respond to the temporal change in phase difference. A neuron being excited by a phase lead, for example, will additionally be driven by a change of the phase in the direction from lag to lead. It is important for the animal to recognize modulations in phase, such as the transition from a phase lag to a phase lead, and by responding to the temporal change of phase, these neurons can still provide the necessary information even if the value of the phase difference is biased by a small offset due to incorrect timing of afferent signals (Rose and Heiligenberg 1986b).

Nervous systems commonly show multiple representations of sensory information and motor control systems. As suggested earlier in connection with the multiple maps of the ELL, multiple representations appear to arise through duplications of existing structures and should facilitate the emergence of new adaptations. To the extent that a given function can be fulfilled by more than one system, the animal can afford the luxury of tinkering with individual systems, and the resulting modifications may prove advantageous for present or future challenges by its environment. The gymnotiform genus *Sternopygus* does not perform a JAR (Bullock et al. 1972), but its torus semicircularis and nucleus electrosensorius contain types of neurons that could readily be hooked up to generate this behavior (Rose et al. 1987). Moreover, this fish can be conditioned to discriminate the sign of a frequency difference between a jamming signal and its own EOD by responding with physical maneuvers (Rose, personal communication). A neuronal network adapted to the electrosensory analysis of moving objects contains a variety of amplitude- and phase-coding neurons that provide the necessary information for the control of the JAR. All that is needed is an appropriate pooling of outputs from neurons coding certain aspects of information and their connection with suitable premotor elements. Individual higher-order neurons of the torus were found to send collaterals to as many as five different targets, tectum, nucleus electrosensorius, dorsal thalamus, nucleus praeeminentialis, and reticular formation; each of these stations is assumed to serve a different behavioral function. It appears plausible that further collaterals and additional behavioral functions could evolve in the future. Indeed, *Sternopygus* is considered the most ancestral gymnotiform (Fink and Fink 1981), and it is likely that the JAR arose in more advanced species from these preexisting electrosensory components.

Yet little is known about developmental rules leading to the correct choice of adaptive behavioral responses. While ordered neuronal maps appear to form even in the absence of sensory experience (Udin and Fawcett 1988), their ultimate shape, as in the case of the primate somatosensory cortex (Merzenich et al. 1987, Recanzone et al. 1989), and the topographic alignment of maps of different modalities within multimodal representations, such as in the superior colliculus of the barn owl (Knudsen and Knudsen 1989, 1990), strongly depend on sensory experience. Hebbian-type rules appear to ensure that jointly activated synapses reinforce each other, and this mechanism may suffice for an ordered separation of pathways and projections, such as those controlling flexion and extension of a muscle. But what remains to be secured is the choice of the correct, adaptive behavioral pattern (e.g., flexion or extension) in response to a specific stimulus configuration. This choice could be achieved by a general reward system which would condition the animal to select the correct behavior, but it could also be determined genetically at the structural level. While the second class of mechanisms appears to be the norm in invertebrates, it has less commonly been demonstrated in vertebrates.

An example is the JAR in *Eigenmannia*. When this behavior emerges in juveniles its correct execution does not require prior experience with interfering signals of neighbors (Hagedorn et al. 1988). Fish raised from the egg stage in isolation lower their electric organ discharge frequency on their first encounter with an interfering signal of slightly higher frequency and raise their own frequency in the case of a signal of slightly lower frequency, provided that they have reached a sufficient size. When exposed to interfering signals at an earlier stage, however, some juveniles may shift their frequency in the wrong direction. Yet these same individuals correct their responses over the course of a few days although they receive no feedback from which to determine the correctness of their responses. These fish are tested exclusively with a signal frequency actively clamped to their own frequency to maintain a given, constant frequency difference, and, therefore, a fish can never succeed in shifting its own frequency away from the interfering signal frequency (Viete 1990; Viete and Heiligenberg 1991). It thus appears that the JAR only requires developmental time sufficient for a complete wiring of its circuitry and that specific sensory experience is unnecessary. This is an example of an innate behavior as envisioned by early ethologists.

References

Allman JM, Kaas JH (1971) A representation of the visual field in the caudal third of the middle temporal gyrus of the owl monkey (*Aotus trivirgatus*). Brain Res 31: 84–105

Allman JM, Kaas JH (1974) A crescent-shaped cortical visual area surrounding the middle temporal area (MT) in the owl monkey (*Aotus trivirgatus*). Brain Res 76: 247–265

Allman JM, Baker JF, Newsome WT, Petersen SE (1981) Visual topography and function. In: Woolsey CN (ed) Cortical Sensory Organization. Humana Press, Clifton, New Jersey, vol. 2: 171–185

Baker CL (1980) Jamming avoidance behavior in gymnotoid electric fish with pulse-type discharges: Sensory coding for a temporal pattern discrimination. J Comp Physiol 136: 165–181

Baker CL (1981) Sensory control of pacemaker acceleration and deceleration in gymnotiform electric fish with pulse-type discharges. J Comp Physiol 141: 197–206

Baldi P, Heiligenberg W (1988) How sensory maps could enhance resolution through ordered arrangements of broadly tuned receivers. Biol Cybern 59: 313–318

Bass AH (1986) Electric organs revisited: Evolution of a vertebrate communication and orientation organ. In: Bullock TH, Heiligenberg W (eds) Electroreception. John Wiley and Sons, New York, pp 13–70

Bass AH, Hopkins CD (1983) Hormonal control of sexual differentiation: Changes in electric organ discharge waveform. Science 220: 971–974

Bass AH, Hopkins CD (1985) Hormonal control of sex differences in the electric organ discharge (EOD) of mormyrid fish. J Comp Physiol A 156: 587–604

Bastian J (1982) Vision and electroreception: Integration of sensory information in the optic tectum of the weakly electric fish *Apteronotus albifrons*. J Comp Physiol 147: 287–297

Bastian J (1986a) Electrolocation: Behavior, anatomy and physiology. In: Bullock TH, Heiligenberg W (eds) Electroreception. Wiley and Sons, New York, pp 577–612

Bastian J (1986b) Gain control in the electrosensory system: A role for the descending projections to the electrosensory lateral line lobe. J Comp Physiol A 158: 505–515

Bastian J, Bratton B (1990) Descending control of electroreception. I: Properties of nucleus praeeminentialis neurons projecting indirectly to the electrosensory lateral line lobe. J Neurosci 10: 1226–1240

Bastian J, Heiligenberg W (1980a) Neural correlates of the jamming avoidance response in *Eigenmannia*. J Comp Physiol 136: 135–152

Bastian J, Heiligenberg W (1980b) Phase sensitive midbrain neurons in *Eigenmannia*: Neural correlates of the jamming avoidance response. Science 209: 828–831

Bastian J, Yuthas J (1984) The jamming avoidance response of *Eigenmannia*: Properties of a diencephalic link between sensory processing and motor output. J Comp Physiol A 154: 895–908

Behrend K (1977) Processing information carried in a high-frequency wave: Properties of cerebellar units in a high-frequency electric fish. J Comp Physiol 118: 357–371

Bekoff A (1986) Ontogeny of chicken motor behaviors: Evidence for multi-use limb pattern generating circuitry. In: Grillner S, Stein PSG, Stuart DG, Frossberg H, Herman RM, Wallen P (eds) Neurobiology of Vertebrate Locomotion. Macmillan, Hampshire/England, pp 433–453

Bekoff A, Nusbaum MP, Sabichi AL, Clifford M (1987) Neural control of limb coordination. I. Comparison of hatching and walking motor output patterns in normal and deafferented chicks. J Neurosci 7: 2320–2330

Bekoff A, Kauer JA, Fulstone A, Summers TR (1989) Neural control of limb coordination. II. Hatching and walking motor output patterns in the absence of input from the brain. Exp Brain Res 74: 609–617

Bell CC (1989) Sensory coding and corollary discharge effects in mormyrid electric fish. J Exp Biol 146: 229–253

Bell CC, Myers JP, Russel CJ (1974) Electric organ discharge patterns during dominance-related behavioral displays in *Gnathonemus petersii*. J Comp Physiol 92: 201–228

Bennett MVL (1971) Electric organs. In: Hoar WS, Randall DJ (eds) Fish Physiology. Academic Press, New York, pp 493–574

Borst A, Egelhaaf M (1989) Principles of visual motion detection. TINS 12: 297–306

Bratton B, Bastian J (1990) Descending control of electroreception. II: Properties of nucleus praeeminentialis neurons projecting directly to the electrosensory lateral line lobe. J Neurosci 10: 1241–1253

Bullock TH (1968) Biological Sensors. In: Vistas in Science. Albuquerque, University of New Mexico

Bullock TH, Chichibu S (1965) Further analysis of sensory coding in electroreceptors of electric fish. Proc Natl Acad Sci USA 54: 422–429

Bullock TH, Heiligenberg W (eds) (1986) Electroreception. John Wiley and Sons, New York

Bullock TH, Hamstra RH, Scheich H (1972) The jamming avoidance response of high-frequency electric fish, I & II. J Comp Physiol 77: 1–48

Bullock TH, Behrend K, Heiligenberg W (1975) Comparison of the jamming avoidance response in gymnotoid and gymnarchid electric fish: A case of convergent evolution of behavior and its sensory basis. J Comp Physiol 103: 97–121

Carr CE, Maler L (1985) A Golgi study of the cell types of the dorsal torus semicircularis of the electric fish *Eigenmannia*: Functional and morphological diversity in the midbrain. J Comp Neurol 235: 207–240

Carr CE, Maler L (1986) Electroreception in gymnotiform fish: Central anatomy and physiology. In: Bullock TH, Heiligenberg W (eds) Electroreception. New York, John Wiley and Sons, pp. 319–374

Carr CE, Maler L, Heiligenberg W, Sas E (1981) Laminar organization of the afferent and efferent systems of the torus semicircularis of gymnotiform fish: Morphological substrates for parallel processing in the electrosensory system. J Comp Neurol 203: 649–670

Carr CE, Maler L, Sas E (1982) Peripheral organization and central projections of the electrosensory nerves in gymnotiform fish. J Comp Neurol 211: 139–153

Carr CE, Heiligenberg W, Rose GJ (1986a) A time-comparison circuit in the electric fish midbrain. I. Behavior and physiology. J Neurosci 6:107–119

Carr CE, Maler L, Taylor B (1986b) A time-comparison circuit in the electric fish midbrain. II. Functional morphology. J Neurosci 6: 1372–1383

Choongkil L, Rohrer WH, Sparks DL (1988) Population coding of saccadic eye movements by neurons in the superior colliculus. Nature 332: 357–360

Crews D (1975) Effects of different components of male courtship behavior on environmentally induced ovarian recrudescence and mating preferences in the lizard *Anolis carolinensis*. Anim Behav 23: 347–356

Crick F (1984) Function of the thalamic reticular complex: The searchlight hypothesis. Proc Natl Acad Sci USA 81: 4586–4590

DeYoe EA, van Essen DC (1988) Concurrent processing streams in monkey visual cortex. TINS 11: 219–226

Dumont PC, Robertson RM (1986) Neuronal circuits: An evolutionary perspective. Science 233: 849–853

Dye JC (1987) Dynamics and behavioral contexts distinguishing modes of pacemaker modulations in the weakly electric fish *Apteronotus*. J Comp Physiol A 161: 175–185

Dye JC (1988) An in vitro physiological preparation of a vertebrate communicatory behavior: Chirping in the weakly electric fish, *Apteronotus*. J Comp Physiol A 163: 445–458.

Dye JC, Heiligenberg W (1987) Intracellular recording in the medullary pacemaker nucleus of the weakly electric fish, *Apteronotus*, during modulatory behaviors. J Comp Physiol A 161: 187–200

Dye JC, Meyer JH (1986) Central control of the electric organ discharge in weakly electric fish. In: Bullock TH, Heiligenberg W (eds) Electroreception. John Wiley and Sons, New York, pp 71–102

Dye JC, Heiligenberg W, Keller C, Kawasaki M (1989) Different classes of glutamate receptors mediate distinct behaviors in a single brainstem nucleus. Proc Natl Acad Sci USA 86: 8993–8997

Ewert JP (1987) Neuroethology of releasing mechanisms: Prey catching in toads. Behav Brain Sci 10: 337–405

Finger TE, Bell CC, Carr CE (1986) Why are electrosensory systems so similar? In: Bullock TH, Heiligenberg W (eds) Electroreception. John Wiley and Sons, New York, pp 465–481

Fink SV, Fink WL (1981) Interrelationships of the ostariophysan fishes (Teleostei). Zool J Linn Soc 72: 297–353

Georgopoulos AP, Kettner RE, Schwartz AB (1988) Primate motor cortex and free arm movements to visual targets in three-dimensional space. II. Coding of the direction of movement by a neuronal population. J Neurosci 8: 2928–2937

Georgopoulos AP, Lurito JT, Petrides M, Schwartz AB (1989) Mental rotation of the neuronal population vector. Science 243: 234–236

Getting PA (1989a) Emerging principles governing the operation of neural networks. Annu Rev Neurosci 12: 185–204

Getting PA (1989b) A network oscillator underlying swimming in *Tritonia*. In: Jacklett JW (ed) Neuronal and Cellular Oscillators. Marcel Decker, New York, Basel, pp 215–236

Grillner S, Buchanan JT, Wallen P, Brodin L (1988) Neural control of locomotion in lower vertebrates: From behavior to ionic mechanisms. In: Cohen AH, Rossignol S, Grillner S (eds) Neural Control of Rhythmic Movements in Vertebrates. John Wiley and Sons, New York, pp 1–40

Hagedorn M (1986) The ecology, courtship, and mating of gymnotiform electric fish. In: Bullock TH, Heiligenberg W (eds) Electroreception. John Wiley and Sons, New York, pp 497–525

Hagedorn M, Heiligenberg W (1985) Court and spark: Electric signals in the courtship and mating of gymnotoid electric fish. Anim Behav 33: 254–265

Hagedorn M, Heiligenberg W, Carr CE (1988) The development of the jamming avoidance response in the weakly electric fish *Eigenmannia*. Brain Behav Evol 31: 161–169

Harris-Warrick RM, Marder EE (1991) Modulation of neural networks for behavior. Annu Rev Neurosci 14: 39–57

Heiligenberg W (1973) Electrolocation of objects in the electric fish *Eigenmannia* (Rhamphichthyidae, Gymnotoidei). J Comp Physiol 87: 137–164

Heiligenberg W (1974) Electrolocation and jamming avoidance in a *Hypopygus* (Rhamphichthyidae, Gymnotoidei), an electric fish with pulse-type discharges. J Comp Physiol 91: 223–240

Heiligenberg W (1975) Electrolocation and jamming avoidance in the electric fish *Gymnarchus niloticus*. J Comp Physiol 103: 55–67

Heiligenberg W (1976) Electrolocation and jamming avoidance in the mormyrid fish *Brienomyrus*. J Comp Physiol 109: 357–372

Heiligenberg W (1977a) Principles of Electrolocation and Jamming Avoidance. Studies of Brain Function. Vol 1. Springer Verlag, Berlin-Heidelberg-New York, pp 1–85

Heiligenberg W (1977b) Releasing and motivating functions of stimulus patterns in animal behavior: The ends of a spectrum. In: Wenzel BM, Zeigler HP (eds) Tonic Functions of Sensory Systems. Annals of the New York Academy of Science, 290: 60–71, New York Academy of Science, New York

Heiligenberg W (1980) The jamming avoidance response in the weakly electric fish *Eigenmannia*. Naturwissenschaften 67: 499–507

Heiligenberg W (1986) Jamming avoidance responses, model systems for neuroethology. In: Bullock TH, Heiligenberg W (eds) Electroreception. John Wiley and Sons, New York, pp 613–649

Heiligenberg W (1987) Central processing of sensory information in electric fish. J Comp Physiol A 161: 621–631

Heiligenberg W (1989) Coding and processing of electrosensory information in gymnotiform fish. J Exp Biol 146: 255–275

Heiligenberg W (1991) The neural basis of behavior: A neuroethological view. Annu Rev Neurosci 14: 247–267

Heiligenberg W, Bastian J (1980) The control of *Eigenmannia's* pacemaker by distributed evaluation of electroreceptive afferences. J Comp Physiol 136: 113–133

Heiligenberg W, Dye JC (1982) Labelling of electroreceptive afferents in gymnotoid fish by intracellular injection of HRP: The mystery of multiple maps. J Comp Physiol A 148: 287–296

Heiligenberg W, Partridge BL (1981) How electroreceptors encode JAR-eliciting stimulus regimes: Reading trajectories in a phase-amplitude plane. J Comp Physiol 142: 295–308

Heiligenberg W, Rose GJ (1985) Phase and amplitude computations in the midbrain of an electric fish: Intracellular studies of neurons participating in the jamming avoidance response of *Eigenmannia*. J Neurosci 2: 515–531

Heiligenberg W, Rose GJ (1986) Gating of sensory information: Joint computations of phase and amplitude data in the midbrain of the electric fish *Eigenmannia*. J Comp Physiol 159: 311–324

Heiligenberg W, Rose GJ (1987) The optic tectum of the gymnotiform electric fish *Eigenmannia*: Labelling of physiologically identified cells. Neuroscience 22: 331–340

Heiligenberg W, Baker C, Bastian J (1978a) The jamming avoidance response in gymnotoid pulse species: A mechanism to minimize the probability of pulse-train coincidences. J Comp Physiol 124: 211–224

Heiligenberg W, Baker C, Matsubara J (1978b) The jamming avoidance response in *Eigenmannia* revisited: The structure of a neuronal democracy. J Comp Physiol 127: 267–286

Heiligenberg W, Finger T, Matsubara J, Carr CE (1981) Input to the medullary pacemaker nucleus in the weakly electric fish, *Eigenmannia* (Sternopygidae, Gymnotiformes). Brain Res 211: 418–423

Heiligenberg W, Keller CH, Metzner W, Kawasaki M (1991) Structure and function of neurons in the complex of the nucleus electrosensorius of the gymnotiform fish *Eigenmannia*: Detection and processing of electric signals in social communication. J Comp Physiol A (in press)

Hopkins CD (1972) Sex differences in electric signalling in an electric fish. Science 176: 1035–1037

Hopkins CD (1973) Lightening as a background noise for communication among electric fish. Nature 242: 286–270

Hopkins CD (1974a) Electric communication in fish. Am Scientist 62: 426–437

Hopkins CD (1974b) Electric communication: Functions in the social behavior of *Eigenmannia virescens*. Behavior 50 (3–4): 270–305

Hopkins CD (1974c) Electric communication in the reproductive behavior of *Sternopygus macrurus* (Gymnotoidei). Zeitschr Tierpsychol 35: 518–535

Hopkins CD (1976) Stimulus filtering and electroreception: Tuberous electroreceptors in three species of gymnotoid fish. J Comp Physiol 111: 171–208

Hopkins CD (1980) Evolution of electric communication channels of mormyrids. Behav Ecol Sociobiol 7:1–13

Hopkins CD (1986) Behavior of mormyridae. In: Bullock TH, Heiligenberg W (eds) Electroreception. Wiley and Sons, New York, pp 527–576

Hopkins CD (1988) Neuroethology of electric communication. Ann Rev Neurosci 11: 497–535

Horikawa K, Armstrong WE (1988) A versatile mean of intracellular labeling: Injection of biocytin and its detection with avidin conjugates. J Neurosci Methods 25:1–12

Hoy R, Nolen T, Brodfuehrer P (1989) The neuroethology of acoustic startle and escape in flying insects. J Exp Biol 146: 287–306

Johnston SA, Maler L (1989) Carbocyanine dye labelled neurons and processes of Apteronotus leptorhynchus projecting to the pituitary neurochemical identity. Society for Neuroscience, Abstr. 454.15

Kalmijn AJ (1984) Theory of electromagnetic orientation: A further analysis. In: Bolis L, Keynes RD, Maddrell SHP (eds) Comparative Physiology of Sensory Systems. Cambridge University Press, Cambridge, pp 525–560

Kalmijn AJ (1987) Detection of weak electric fields. In: Atema J, Fay RR, Popper AN, Tavolga WN (eds) Sensory Biology of Aquatic Animals. Springer Verlag, Berlin-Heidelberg-New York, pp 151–186

Katz PS, Harris-Warrick RM (1990) Actions of identified neuromodulatory neurons in a simple motor system. TINS 13: 367–373

Karten HJ, Shimizu T (1990) The origins of neocortex: Connections and lamination as distinct events in evolution. J Cog Neurosci 1(4): 291–301

Kawasaki M, Heiligenberg W (1988) Individual prepacemaker neurons can modulate the medullary pacemaker of the gymnotiform electric fish, Eigenmannia. J Comp Physiol A 162: 13–21

Kawasaki M, Heiligenberg W (1989) Distinct mechanisms of modulation in a neuronal oscillator generate different social signals in the electric fish Hypopomus. J Comp Physiol A 165: 731–741

Kawasaki M, Heiligenberg W (1990) Different classes of glutamate receptors and GABA mediate distinct modulations of a neuronal oscillator, the medullary pacemaker of a gymnotiform electric fish. J Neurosci 10(12): 3896–3904

Kawasaki M, Maler L, Rose GJ, Heiligenberg W (1988a) Anatomical and functional organization of the prepacemaker nucleus in gymnotiform electric fish: The accommodation of two behaviors in one nucleus. J Comp Neurol 276: 113–131

Kawasaki M, Rose GJ, Heiligenberg W (1988b) Temporal hyperacuity in single neurons of electric fish. Nature 336: 173–176

Keller CH (1988) Stimulus discrimination in the diencephalon of Eigenmannia: The emergence and sharpening of a sensory filter. J Comp Physiol A 162: 747–757

Keller CH, Heiligenberg W (1989) From distributed sensory processing to discrete motor representations in the diencephalon of the electric fish, Eigenmannia. J Comp Physiol A 164: 565–576

Keller CH, Kawasaki M, Heiligenberg W (1989) Intracellular labelling of physiologically identified cells within a diencephalic sensory-motor interface. Society for Neuroscience, Abstr. 454.5

Keller CH, Maler L, Heiligenberg W (1990) Structural and functional organization of a diencephalic sensory-motor interface in the gymnotiform fish, *Eigenmannia*. J Comp Neurol 293: 347–376

Kirschbaum F (1983) Myogenic electric organ precedes the neurogenic organ in apteronotid fish. Naturwissenschaften 70: 205–207

Knudsen EI, Knudsen PF (1989) Vision calibrates sound localization in developing barn owls. J Neurosci 9: 3306–3313

Knudsen EI, Knudsen PF (1990) Sensitive and critical periods for visual calibration of sound localization by barn owls. J. Neurosci 10: 222–232

Konishi M (1986) Centrally synthesized maps of sensory space. TINS 9: 163–168

Konishi M (1991) Deciphering the brain's code. Neural Computation 3: 1–18

Konishi M, Takahashi TT, Wagner H, Sullivan WE, Carr CE (1988) Neurophysiological and anatomical substrates of sound localization in the owl. In: Edelman GM, Gall WE, Cowan WM (eds) Auditory Function. John Wiley and Sons, New York, pp 721–745

Kramer B (1974) Electric organ discharge interaction during interspecific agonistic behavior in freely swimming mormyrid fish. A method to evaluate two or more. J Comp Physiol 93: 203–236

Kramer B (1985) Jamming avoidance in the electric fish *Eigenmannia*: Harmonic analysis of sexually dimorphic waves. J Exp Biol 119: 41–69

Larimer JL (1988) The command hypothesis: A new view using an old example. TINS 11: 506–512

Lehrer M, Srinivasan MV (1989) Motion detection in the bee as a tool for distance estimation and object discrimination. In: Erber J, Menzel R, Pflüger HJ, Todt D (eds) Neural Mechanisms of Behavior. Georg Thieme Verlag, Stuttgart, pp 234–235

Lehrer M, Srinivasan MV, Zhang SW (1990) Visual edge detection in the honeybee and its chromatic properties. Proc R Soc London B 238: 321–330

Lehrman DC (1965) Interaction between internal and external environments in the regulation of the reproductive cycle of the ring dove. In: Beach F (ed) Sex and Behavior. John Wiley and Sons, New York, pp 355–380

Lissmann HW (1958) On the function and evolution of electric organs in fish. J Exp Biol 35 (1): 156–191

Lissmann HW, Machin KE (1958) The mechanism of object location in *Gymnarchus niloticus* and similar fish. J Exp Biol 35: 451–486

Livingstone MS, Hubel DH (1987) Psychophysical evidence for separate channels for the perception of form, color, movement and depth. J Neurosci 7: 3416–3468

Mago-Leccia F (1978) Los peces de la familia Sternopygidae de Venezuela. Acta Cientifica Venezolana, Vol. 29, Supl. 1, pp 1–89

Maler L, Mugnaini E (1986) Immunohistochemical identification of GABA-ergic synapses in the electrosensory lateral line lobe of a weakly electric fish, *Apteronotus leptorhynchus*. Society for Neuroscience, Abstr. 84: 312

Maler L, Sas E, Rogers J (1981) The cytology of the posterior lateral line lobe of high-frequency weakly electric fish (Gymnotoidei): Dendritic differentiation and synaptic specificity in a simple cortex. J Comp Neurol 195: 87–140

Maler L, Sas E, Carr CE, Matsubara J (1982) Efferent projections of the posterior lateral line lobe in gymnotiform fish. J Comp Neurol 211: 154–164

Maler L, Boland M, Patrick J, Ellis W (1983) Localization of zinc in the pacemaker nucleus of high-frequency gymnotoid fish. In: Frederickson CJ, Howell GA, Kasaroulis EJ (eds) The Neurobiology of Zinc. Part A: Physiochemistry, Anatomy and Techniques. Liss, New York, pp 199–212

Mathieson WB, Maler L (1988) Morphological and electrophysiological properties of a novel in vitro preparation: The electrosensory lateral line lobe brain slice. J Comp Physiol A 163, 489–506.

Mathieson WB, Heiligenberg W, Maler L (1987) Ultrastructural studies of physiologically identified electrosensory afferent synapses in the gymnotiform fish Eigenmannia. J Comp Neurol 255: 526–537

Matsubara JA, Heiligenberg W (1978) How well do electric fish electrolocate under jamming? J Comp Physiol 125: 285–290

Merzenich MM, Nelson RJ, Kaas JH, Strycker MP, Jenkins WM, Zook JM, Cynader MS, Schoppmann A (1987) Variability in hand surface representations in areas 3b and 1 in adult owl and squirrel monkeys. J Comp Neurol 258: 281–96

Metzner W, Heiligenberg W (1990) Neural coding and processing of communicatory signals in the electric fish, *Eigenmannia*. Neuroscience Abstr 548.8, 20th Annual Meeting, St. Louis

Metzner M, Heiligenberg W (1991) The coding of signals in the electric communication of the gymnotiform fish *Eigenmannia*: From electroreceptors to neurons in the torus semicircularis of the midbrain. J Comp Physiol A (in press)

Meyer JH (1984) Steroid influences upon the discharge frequencies of intact and isolated pacemakers of weakly electric fish. J Comp Physiol A 154: 659–668

Moller P (1970) Communication in weakly electric fish, *Gnathonemus niger* (Mormyridae) I. Variation of electric organ discharge (EOD) frequency elicited by controlled electric stimuli. Anim Behav 18: 768–786

Nadi S, Maler L (1987) The laminar distribution of amino acids in the caudal cerebellum and electrosensory lateral line lobe of weakly electric fish (Gymnotidae). Brain Res 425: 218–224

Northcutt RG (1986) Electroreception in non-teleost bony fish. In: Bullock TH, Heiligenberg W (eds) Electroreception. Wiley and Sons, New York, pp 257–285

Partridge BL, Heiligenberg W (1980) Three's a crowd? Predicting *Eigenmannia's* response to multiple jamming. J Comp Physiol 136: 153–164

Partridge BL, Heiligenberg W, Matsubara JA (1981) The neural basis of a sensory filter in the jamming avoidance response: No grandmother cells in sight. J Comp Physiol 145: 153–168

Perret DI, Harries MH, Bevan R, Thomas S, Benson PJ, Mistlin AJ, Chitty AJ, Hietanen JK, Ortega JE (1989) Frameworks of analysis for the neural representation of animate objects and actions. J Exp Biol 146: 87–113

Recanzone GH, Jenkins WM, Hradek GT, Schreiner CE, Graiski KA, Merzenich MM (1989) Frequency discrimination training alters topographical representations and distributed temporal response properties of neurons in S1 cortex of adult owl monkeys. Society for Neuroscience, Abstr. 481.10

Rose GJ, Heiligenberg W (1985a) Structure and function of electrosensory neurons in the torus semicircularis of *Eigenmannia:* Morphological correlates of phase and amplitude sensitivity. J Neurosci 5: 2269–2280

Rose GJ, Heiligenberg W (1985b) Temporal hyperacuity in the electric sense of fish. Nature 318:178–180

Rose GJ, Heiligenberg W (1986a) Neural coding of difference frequencies in the midbrain of the electric fish *Eigenmannia:* Reading the sense of rotation in an amplitude-phase plane. J Comp Physiol A 158: 613–624

Rose GJ, Heiligenberg W (1986b) Limits of phase and amplitude sensitivity in the torus semicircularis of *Eigenmannia.* J Comp Physiol A 159: 813–822

Rose GJ, Keller CH, Heiligenberg W (1987) "Ancestral" neural mechanisms of electrolocation suggest a substrate for the evolution of the jamming avoidance response. J Comp Physiol A 160: 491–500

Rose GJ, Kawasaki M, Heiligenberg W (1988) "Recognition units" at the top of a neuronal hierarchy? J Comp Physiol A 162: 759–772.

Rowell CHF (1989) Descending interneurones of the locust reporting deviation from flight course: What is their role in steering. J Exp Biol 146: 177–194

Sas E, Maler L (1983) The nucleus praeeminentialis: A Golgi study of a feedback center in the electrosensory system of gymnotoid fish. J Comp Neurol 221: 127–144

Saunders J, Bastian J (1984) The physiology and morphology of two types of electrosensory neurons in the weakly electric fish *Apteronotus leptorhynchus*. J Comp Physiol A 154: 199–209

Scheich H (1974) Neural analysis of wave form in the time domain: Midbrain units in electric fish during social behavior. Science 185: 365–367

Scheich H (1977) Neural basis of communication in the high-frequency electric fish *Eigenmannia virescens* (jamming avoidance response). J Comp Physiol 113: 181–255

Scheich H, Bullock TH (1974) The role of electroreceptors in the animal's life. II. The detection of electric fields from electric organs. In: Fessard A (ed) Handbook of Sensory Physiology, Vol. III/3. Springer Verlag, Berlin-Heidelberg-New York, pp 201–256

Scheich H, Ebbesson SOE (1981) Inputs to the torus semicircularis in the electric fish *Eigenmannia virescens*. Cell Tissue Res 215: 531–536

Scheich H, Ebbesson SOE (1983) Multimodal torus in the weakly electric fish *Eigenmannia*. In: Advances in Anatomy, Embryology and Cell Biology, Vol. 82, pp. 1–69. Springer Verlag, Berlin.

Scheich H, Bullock TH, Hamstra RH (1973) Coding properties of two classes of afferent nerve fibers: High-frequency electroreceptors in the electric fish, *Eigenmannia*. J Neurophysiol 36: 39–60

Scheich H, Gottschalk B, Nickel B (1977) The jamming avoidance response in *Rhamphichthys rostratus:* An alternative principle of time domain analysis in electric fish. Exp Brain Res 28: 229–233

Schildberger K (1989) Acoustic communication in crickets: Neural mechanisms of song pattern recognition and sound localization. In: Erber J, Menzel R, Pflüger HJ, Todt D (eds) Neural Mechanisms of Behavior. Georg Thieme Verlag, Stuttgart, 84–89

Shumway CA (1989a) Multiple electrosensory maps in the medulla of weakly electric gymnotiform fish. I. Physiological differences. J Neurosci 9: 4388–4399

Shumway CA (1989b) Multiple electrosensory maps in the medulla of weakly electric gymnotiform fish. II. Anatomical differences. J Neurosci 9: 4400–4415

Shumway CA, Maler L (1989) GABAergic inhibition shapes temporal and spatial response properties of pyramidal cells in the electrosensory lateral line lobe of gymnotoid fish. J Comp Physiol A 164: 391–407.

Simmons JA (1973) The resolution of target range by echolocating bats. J Acoust Soc Am 54: 157–173

Sparks DL (1986) Translation of sensory signals into commands for control of saccadic eye movements: Role of primate superior colliculus. Physiol Rev 66: 118–171

Sparks DL (1988) Neuronal cartography: Sensory and motor maps in the superior colliculus. Brain Behav Evol 31: 49–56

Sparks DL (1989) The neural coding of the location of targets for saccadic eye movements. J Exp Biol 146: 195–207

Sparks DL, Mays LE (1990) Signal transformations required for the generation of saccadic eye movements. Annu Rev Neurosci 13: 309–336

Srinivasan MV, Lehrer M, Horridge GA (1990) Visual figure-ground discrimination in the honeybee: The role of motion parallax at boundaries. Proc R Soc London B 238: 331–350

Stein PSG, Mortin LI, Robertson GA (1986) The forms of a task and their blends. In: Grillner S, Stein PSG, Stuart DG, Frossberg H, Herman RM, Wallen P (eds) Neurobiology of Vertebrate Locomotion. Macmillan, Hampshire/England, pp 201–216

Suga N (1984) The extent to which biosonar information is represented in the bat auditory cortex. In: Edelman GM, Gall WE, Cowan WM (eds) Dynamic Aspects of Neocortical Function. John Wiley and Sons, New York, pp 315–373

Suga N (1988a) Auditory neuroethology and speech processing: Complex-sound processing by combination-sensitive neurons. In: Edelman GM, Gall WE, Cowan WM (eds) Auditory Function. John Wiley and Sons, New York, pp 679–720,

Suga N (1988b) What does single-unit analysis in the auditory cortex tell us about information processing in the auditory system? In: Rakic P, Singer W (eds) Neurobiology of Neocortex. John Wiley and Sons, New York, pp 331–349

Suga N, Horikawa J (1986) Multiple time axes for representation of echo delays in the auditory cortex of the mustached bat. J Neurophysiol 55: 776–805

Szabo T, Heiligenberg W, Ravaille-Veron M (1989) HRP labeling and ultrastructural localization of prepacemaker terminals within the medullary pacemaker nucleus of the weakly electric gymnotiform fish *Apteronotus leptorhynchus*. J Comp Neurol 824: 169–173

Takahashi T (1989) The neural coding of auditory space. J Exp Biol 146: 307–322

Udin SB, Fawcett JW (1988) Formation of topographic maps. Annu Rev Neurosci 11: 289–327

Viete S (1990) The development of the jamming avoidance response (JAR) in *Eigenmannia*: Behavioral and anatomical aspects. Diploma Thesis in Biology, University of Tübingen, Germany

Viete S, Heiligenberg W (1991) The development of the Jamming Avoidance Response (JAR) in *Eigenmannia*: An innate behavior indeed. J Comp Physiol A (in press)

Wehner R (1989a) Neurobiology of polarization vision. TINS 12(9): 353–359

Wehner R (1989b) The hymenopteran skylight compass: Matched filtering and parallel coding. J Exp Biol 146: 63–85

Watanabe A, Takeda K (1963) The change of discharge frequency by A.C. stimulus in a weakly electric fish. J Exp Biol 40: 57–66

Waxman SG, Pappas GD, Bennett MVL (1972) Morphological correlates of functional differentiation of nodes of Ranvier along single fibers in the neurogenic electric organ of the knife fish, *Sternarchus*. J Cell Biol 53: 210–224

Westheimer G, McKee SP (1977) Spatial configurations for hyperacuity. Vision Res 17: 941–947

Wingfield JC (1985) Short-term changes in plasma levels of hormones during establishment and defense of a breeding territory in male song sparrows, *Melospiza melodia*. Horm Behav 19: 174–187

Wingfield JC, Marler P (1988) Endocrine basis of communication in reproduction and aggression. In: Knobil E, Neill J (eds) The Physiology of Reproduction. Raven Press, New York, pp 1647–1677

Wingfield JC, Moore MC (1987) Hormonal, social and environmental factors in the reproductive biology of free-living male birds. In: Crews D (ed) Psychobiology of Reproductive Behavior: An Evolutionary Perspective. Prentice Hall, New Jersey, 148–175

Yuthas J (1985) Motor patterns evoked by stimulation of the optic tectum in two species of weakly electric fish. Society for Neuroscience, Abstr. 300.6

Zakon HH (1986) The electroreceptive periphery. In: Bullock TH, Heiligenberg W (eds) Electroreception. John Wiley and Sons, New York, pp 103–156

Index

Note: Page numbers in *italics* indicate figures.

Printed in the United States
by Baker & Taylor Publisher Services